Patient Encounters

The Neurology and Psychiatry Work-Up

Michael Levy, MD, PhD

Department of Neurology
Johns Hopkins University
Baltimore, Maryland

Series Editor

Alfa O. Diallo, MD, MPH

Department of Emergency Medicine
Johns Hopkins Hospital
Baltimore, Maryland

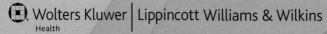
Wolters Kluwer | Lippincott Williams & Wilkins
Health
Philadelphia • Baltimore • New York • London
Buenos Aires • Hong Kong • Sydney • Tokyo

Acquisitions Editor: Susan Rhyner
Product Manager: Stacey L. Sebring
Marketing Manager: Christen Melcher
Compositor: Aptara, Inc.

Copyright © 2010 Lippincott Williams & Wilkins
351 West Camden Street
Baltimore, Maryland 21201-2436 USA
530 Walnut Street
Philadelphia, PA 19106

Printed in the United States of America

Library of Congress Cataloging-in-Publication Data

Levy, Michael, 1975-
  Patient encounters. The neurology and psychiatry work-up / Michael Levy.
     p. ; cm.
  Includes bibliographical references and index.
  ISBN 978-0-7817-9397-1 (alk. paper)
  1. Neurology—Handbooks, manuals, etc. 2. Psychiatry—Handbooks, manuals, etc. 3. Clinical clerkship—Handbooks, manuals, etc. I. Title. II. Title: Psychiatry and neurology work-up.
  [DNLM: 1. Nervous System Diseases—diagnosis. 2. Nervous System Diseases—therapy. 3. Mental Disorders—diagnosis. 4. Mental Disorders—therapy. 5. Neurologic Examination. WL 141 L6675p 2010]
  RC346.L46 2010
  616.8'0475—dc22   2009034623

The publishers have made every effort to trace the copyright holders for borrowed material. If they have inadvertently overlooked any, they will be pleased to make the necessary arrangements at the first opportunity.

We'd like to hear from you! If you have comments or suggestions regarding this Lippincott Williams & Wilkins title, please contact us at the appropriate customer service number listed below, or send correspondence to **book_comments@lww.com**. If possible, please remember to include your mailing address, phone number, and a reference to the book title and author in your message. To purchase additional copies of this book call our customer service department at **(800) 638-3030** or fax orders to **(301) 824-7390**. International customers should call **(301) 714-2324**.

This book is dedicated to all the students on the neurology service at the Johns Hopkins Hospital.

Contributors

Ari M. Blitz, MD
Assistant Professor, Neuroradiology
Russell H. Morgan Dept. of Radiology
and Radiological Science
Johns Hopkins University
Baltimore, Maryland

Joshua B. Ewen, MD
Instructor
Department of Neurology
Johns Hopkins University
Baltimore, Maryland
Director
Clinical Neurophysiology Laboratory
Kennedy Krieger Institute
Baltimore, Maryland

Christina S. Hines, MD, PhD
Housestaff
Department of Psychiatry
Johns Hopkins Hospital
Baltimore, Maryland

Robert E. Hoesch, MD, PhD
Assistant Professor of Neurology and
Fellow in Neurosciences Critical Care
Johns Hopkins University
Baltimore, Maryland

Tyler G. Jones, MD
Forensic Psychiatry Fellow
Department of Psychiatry
Georgetown University Hospital
Washington, DC

George P. Kuo, MD
Resident
Russell H. Morgan Department of
Radiology and Radiological Science
Johns Hopkins Hospital
Baltimore, Maryland

Michael Levy, MD, PhD
Assistant Professor
Department of Neurology
Johns Hopkins University
Baltimore, Maryland

Jeffrey A. Rumbaugh, MD, PhD
Assistant Professor
Department of Neurology
Johns Hopkins University
Baltimore, Maryland

Katherine P. Thomas, MD
Resident Physician
Department of Neurology
Johns Hopkins Hospital
Baltimore, Maryland

Robin K. Wilson, MD, PhD
Associate Director, Adult
Hydrocephalus Center
Sinai Neurology Associates
Sinai Hospital
Baltimore, Maryland

Steven R. Zeiler, MD, PhD
Fellow, Cerebrovascular
The Johns Hopkins Hospital
Baltimore, Maryland

Reviewers

Daniel E. Gih, MD
University of Michigan

Olga Goldberg
Harbor UCLA Medical Center

Jennifer Goldman
SUNY Downstate College of Medicine

Lee Lin, DO
Keck School of Medicine
LAC+USC Medical Center

Ahmed Mian
University of Ottawa Faculty of
Medicine

Vimal Ramjee
Mount Sinai School of Medicine

Stephanie C. Smith, MD
University of Minnesota

Javeed Sukhera, MD
University of Rochester Medical Center

Debra Yerike, MD, MPH
St. Matthew's University School of
Medicine

Preface

The *Patient Encounters* series has been developed to provide a concise review of patient assessment and management. Each book in this series is organized logically and provides medical students with specialty-specific steps for managing patient care. The goal of this series is to remove the focus from "acing the shelf" to a focus on helping medical students become good doctors.

The books in this series provide a specialty-specific, step-by-step guide for managing a patient by candidly addressing, in a very practical fashion, a new clinical clerk's anxiety as well as hunger for learning. Each title within this series is a companion guide that candidly cuts to need-to-know information, directing medical students to what they need to do in each step of the patient encounter.

The books in this series discuss patient care from an overview of the disease or disorder, with brief pathophysiology information presented as necessary to support optimal patient assessment and care. It includes specific information that will help medical students from the point of reviewing the patient's chart to walking into the room and assessing the stability of the patient, including potential life threats. Each book then addresses acute management and workup, directing the student through the diagnosis, treatment, extended inhospital management, and discharge goals and outpatient care.

Each title provides students with the rationale for ordering appropriate diagnostic studies and allows clinical decision making that is consistent with the patient's disposition. The books provide an extended view of patient care so that the medical student can propose a well-informed choice of diagnostic studies and interventions when presenting his or her case to house staff and faculty.

The books use algorithms, tables, figures, icons, and a stylized design to support concise and easy-to-find patient management information. They also provide diagnosis-based, evidence-based information that includes peer-reviewed journal references.

Feedback from student reviewers gives high praise to this new series. Each of these new books was developed to provide practical information and to address the basics needed during a particular clinical rotation:

Patient Encounters: The Inpatient Pediatrics Work-Up
Patient Encounters: The Obstetrics and Gynecology Work-Up
Patient Encounters: The Internal Medicine Work-Up

How to Use This Book

Patient Encounters: The Neurology and Psychiatry Work-Up provides you with a concise, organized review of the most important patient assessment and management in neurology and neuropsychiatry. This book is designed for you to quickly and efficiently review and enhance the knowledge you need to effectively manage patient care.

This book can help you ease the transition from the basic sciences to clinical medicine by providing you with a practical "how-to" guide for approaching a patient, including:

- Identifying pertinent positives and negatives in the patient history and physical exam
- Determining how to work up a patient by addressing pertinent diagnostic studies and procedures
- Explaining the rationale for clinical decision making

The 15 chapters in this text are divided into two sections. Each chapter features essential information related to patient assessment and management, supplemented with patient case studies that provide you with the opportunity to apply patient care principles and management goals to patient cases that are specific to each chapter's topic.

This book, as with all the books in the series, includes common features that will allow you to glean necessary information quickly and easily:

- **The Patient Encounter:** Each chapter begins with a patient case study that is followed up on at several intervals throughout the chapter. The patient encounter allows you the opportunity to see some of the common signs and symptoms with which a patient may present.
- **Overview:** This section provides an introduction to the chapter topic and includes the definition, epidemiology, and etiology of the disease or disorder. Brief pathophysiology information is included to support optimal patient assessment and care.
- **Acute Management and Workup:** This section includes the key information that you need to obtain in order to provide excellent patient care, addressing first what you need to do within the first 15 minutes through the first few hours. Topics include the initial assessment, admission and level of care criteria, the patient history, the physical examination, labs and imaging to consider, and key treatment information.
- **Extended Inhospital Management:** This section provides information that you need to know when a patient needs extended inhospital management.

- **Disposition:** In this section, you will find the key discharge goals and outpatient care related to a patient with the specific condition or disorder addressed in the chapter.
- **What You Need to Remember:** This feature is a bulleted list of key points that are most helpful to remember about the chapter topic.
- **Suggested Readings:** Each chapter provides diagnosis- and evidence-based peer-reviewed journal references.
- **Clinical Pearl:** This feature presents clinical tips, statistics, or findings that will help you understand the patient's clinical presentation or help you better address diagnosis and management.

In addition to the features noted above, this text contains tables, line drawings, and photographs to supplement your learning.

Remember that your team is expecting to get a snapshot of what the patient's disease process is and what we are going to do about it. Therefore, you need to present a "one-liner"—a one-line summary that includes the patient's age, brief past medical history, and his initial clinical symptoms. For example, a one-line summary might be the following: *Ms. Pennypacker is a 78-year-old woman with a history of atrial fibrillation who presents with acute onset of right arm weakness.* You should also provide the relevant history of symptoms, the time of onset, its progression, and any associated symptoms. Summarize the examination, including the pertinent positives and negatives. This is difficult early on because you may not know what is pertinent. Try to be logical—your senior residents and attendings are going through the same process that you went through to figure out the disease. Therefore, give them the information that you thought was important. For instance, *The patient was not dysarthric, he had no cranial nerve abnormalities, but he could not name, could not repeat, was not fluent, but could comprehend.*

Finally, present your assessment. More than anything else, your clear and well-thought out assessment will get you bonus points on a Neurology Clerkship. In presenting your assessment, localize the lesion: Is this a primary problem of speech (phonation or articulation), language (Broca's, Wernicke's, etc.), or cognition? Then state what you think caused the problem (e.g., stroke versus seizure), how we are going to make the diagnosis (e.g., imaging or EEG), and what therapeutic plan we are going to institute.

I hope this text improves your knowledge of neurology and neuropsychiatry, allowing you to feel confident that you're providing quality patient care. The ultimate goal of this book is to better prepare you to provide effective care to patients who you will encounter in your medical career.

Michael Levy, MD, PhD
Department of Neurology
Johns Hopkins University
Baltimore, Maryland

Contents

SECTION 2: Neuropsychiatry

Localization and the Neurological Exam

Neurologists think differently from other doctors. To succeed on your neurology clerkship, you need to learn to think like a neurologist.

WHERE'S THE LESION?

Localization is the single most important skill to learn on your neurology clerkship. The nervous system stretches from the brain to the toe, and dysfunction can occur at many points along way. The first goal in working up a patient in neurology is to localize the dysfunction.

There are eight levels of the nervous system (Fig. 1-1). Each level is characterized by certain anatomic and functional properties that co-localize it.

Level 1

The cerebral cortex is involved in many aspects of motor and sensory function, including vision, memory, language, and higher cognition. Lesions of the cortex can be localized or diffuse. The dysfunction caused by a localized lesion in the cortex depends on the location (Table 1-1), whereas diffuse lesions generally cause altered mental status.

Level 2

The subcortical white matter, which carries myelinated axons between the cortices and other parts of the central nervous system, has three unique properties that help to localize lesions to this area:

1. Small lesions in the subcortical white matter can cause big problems as axons from large areas of the cortex are bundled tightly, coursing down toward the brainstem.
2. Widespread involvement of the subcortical white matter can lead to cognitive impairments *with* motor deficits, especially in gait.
3. Acute weakness and/or numbness of the face, arm, and leg on one side in an awake patient commonly localizes to the contralateral subcortical area.

Medical students often have difficulty distinguishing between cortical and subcortical lesions. Cortical lesions include dysfunction unique to the cortex, such as vision, higher cognitive functions, memory, language, and lateral eye movements. For example, a lesion in the cortex of the left frontal lobe usually affects *both* language production *and* motor activity on the right

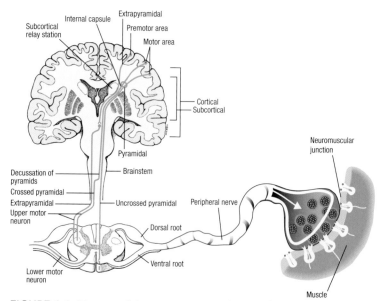

FIGURE 1-1: Diagram of the nervous system showing the eight layers of localization: cortex, subcortex, brainstem, spinal cord, nerve root, peripheral nerve, neuromuscular junction, and muscle.

side of the body. In contrast, right-sided weakness in the setting of *normal* language production makes localization to the cortex less likely.

Level 3

The brainstem includes the thalamus, the midbrain, the pons, and the medulla. When patients present with cranial nerve findings, brainstem involvement should be suspected. The following signs alert you to consider localization to the brainstem: dysconjugate horizontal eye movements; crossed findings involving weakness/numbness of the ipsilateral face and contralateral body; nausea, lightheadedness, or vertigo. Table 1-1 lists the functions of each part of the brainstem, and Figure 1-2 shows the gross anatomic layout of the brain and brainstem (Levels 1–3).

Level 4

Lesions of the spinal cord should be considered when a patient complains of weakness/numbness below the neck, especially when associated with bowel/bladder dysfunction. "Sensory levels," which are characterized by sensory dysfunction below a vertebral level and normal sensation above that vertebral level, almost always localize to the spinal cord. A sensory level at

TABLE 1-1
CNS Function Localization

Brain Region	Loss of Function
Frontal poles	Personality changes; poor executive planning; disinhibited behavior; emotional incontinence.
Left frontal lobe	Eyes deviate to the left; weakness in the right face, arm, leg; motor aphasia (if patient is right-handed).
Right frontal lobe	Eyes deviate to the right; weakness in the left face, arm, leg.
Left parietal lobe	Sensory loss in the right face, arm, leg; sensory aphasia (if patient is right-handed); difficulty with drawing, calculations; right visual field loss.
Right parietal lobe	Sensory loss in the left face, arm, leg; apraxia; left-sided neglect; left visual field loss.
Occipital poles	Vision loss, visual field loss, visual hallucinations.
Brainstem	
Thalamus	Contralateral loss of sensory function; bilateral thalamic lesions can result in loss of consciousness.
Midbrain	Dysfunction of vertical eye movements and pupillary function; contralateral face/arm/leg weakness and sensory loss.
Pons	Dysfunction of lateral eye movements; vestibular dysfunction such as vertigo; crossed findings of ipsilateral face and contralateral arm/leg weakness and sensory loss.
Medulla	Dysfunction of swallowing, autonomic function, and tongue movement.

(continued)

TABLE 1-1
CNS Function Localization (Continued)

Brain Region	Loss of Function
Spinal Cord	
Cervical cord	High cervical lesions affect breathing (C3–C5). Low cervical lesions cause flaccid weakness/sensory loss in arms (C5–C8). Cervical lesions also can cause upper motor neuron signs in the trunk and legs and spastic bladder incontinence.
Thoracic cord	Loss of tone in trunk causes pain and unsteadiness, upper motor neurons signs in the legs and spastic bladder incontinence. May affect autonomic functions such as blood pressure and heart rate control.
Lumbar	Flaccid weakness of the legs. Atonic bladder.

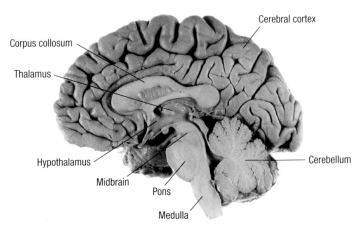

FIGURE 1-2: Midline sagittal view of the brain showing the cerebral cortex, cerebellum, corpus collosum, thalamus, hypothalamus, and three components of the brainstem: midbrain, pons, and medulla. Adapted from Haines, DE. *Neuroanatomy: An Atlas of Structures, Sections, and Systems*, 6th Ed. Lippincott Williams & Wilkins, 2004.

the nipples corresponds to a T4 lesion (or higher); a sensory level at the umbilicus corresponds to a T10 lesion (or higher).

CLINICAL PEARL

When a lesion of the central nervous system is suspected, including cortical, subcortical, brainstem, and spinal cord, look for signs of asymmetric upper motor neuron dysfunction. The two important upper motor neuron signs are hyperflexia and increased tone. If the lesion is above the decussation of the pyramids of the medulla oblongata, the upper motor neuron signs will be contralateral to the lesion. If the lesion is below the decussation (i.e., the spinal cord), the upper neuron signs will be ipsilateral to the lesion.

Level 5

Spinal roots are made up of axons that carry motor impulses from the spinal cord to the muscle and sensory information from the limbs to the spinal cord. The roots are located just outside of the spinal cord but within the vertebral column and are commonly affected by pathology of the vertebrae. They are characterized by their distribution (Fig. 1-3). Lesions of the spinal roots affect only their particular distribution and not any others. For example, dysfunction of the C5 cervical root can cause weakness and numbness in the ipsilateral shoulder area but not in any other cervical or thoracic distributions above or below C5.

CLINICAL PEARL

It is important to differentiate between lesions of the spinal cord and nerve root. Lesions in the spinal cord usually affect sensory and/or motor functions at and below a level, whereas spinal root lesions affect sensory and/or motor function at only one level. In addition, lesions of the spinal cord will result in upper motor neuron signs of hyperreflexia and increased tone in the ipsilateral limbs below the lesion, whereas lesions of the nerve root result in lower motor neuron signs at the affected level only.

Level 6

The nerves between the spinal roots and the muscle are referred to as peripheral nerves. Lesions of the peripheral nerves can occur within individual

Cutaneous areas of peripheral nerve innervation

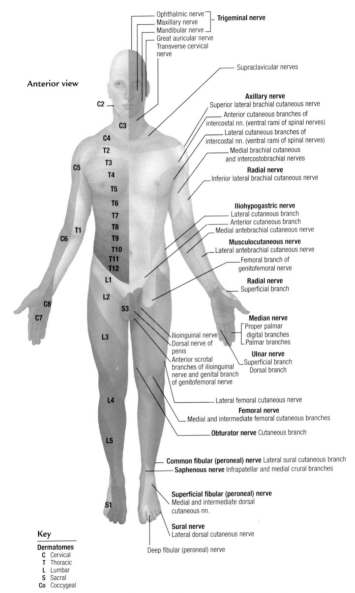

FIGURE 1-3: Human body showing the nerve root distributions and sensory dermatomes. Courtesy of Anatomical Chart Co.

nerves to cause palsies such as radial nerve palsy; they can also occur within bundles such as brachial plexus to affect multiple downstream targets. Localized peripheral nerve lesions (e.g., compression) affect only the muscle and/or sensory area distal to the injury. Diffuse peripheral nerve disease (e.g., diabetic neuropathy) affects the longest nerves first, including the feet and hands, in a symmetric distribution.

Level 7

In the neuromuscular junction, think myasthenia gravis. Disorders of the neuromuscular junction, such as myasthenia gravis, are chronic and diffuse, with proximal muscles weaker than distal muscles. If there are sensory changes or localized weakness only, disorders of the neuromuscular junction are much *less* likely.

Level 8

Lesions in muscle can cause weakness. They also cause pain and tenderness on palpation. Lesions can be local from trauma, or diffuse, such as in rhabdomyolysis. Laboratory testing and muscle biopsy are very helpful in diagnosing primary muscle lesions.

Lesions involving the lower motor neurons in the spinal cord, nerve root, and peripheral nerve and muscle have four similar characteristics and are called lower motor neuron signs: hyporeflexia, hypotonia, fasciculations, and atrophy.

THE NEUROLOGIC PHYSICAL EXAM

Following a thorough general examination, the neurologic exam provides a great deal of useful information. A full neurologic exam can take hours, but with this guide, you can shorten the exam without missing important details.

The neurologic exam is divided into seven areas:

1. *Mental status.* The goal of the mental status exam is to determine if the cerebral cortex is functioning at baseline. As noted earlier in this chapter, there are many functions of the cerebral cortex, but by asking a few simple questions, you can screen for major problems. A full mental status exam is described later in this chapter and also in Chapter 12, Mood Disorders.

Before performing the mental status exam, make sure your patient is awake! Start with a verbal cue to wake up and open his eyes. If there is no response, try gently shaking the patient awake. You can also try to gently hold open his eyelids. A chest rub or pinch is the next step and, finally, if there is no response to any of those methods, try persistent nail bed pressure with a firm object, such as a reflex hammer.

In your awake patient, start by asking the simplest questions/commands. If the patient cannot answer the question or follow the simplest command, there is no point in continuing to ask more difficult questions and commands.

- *Simplest questions/commands:*
  - "What is your name? What is the date? Where are we?" These three simple questions are the most commonly asked questions in neurology. Ask them slowly and give the patient time to answer.
  - "Close your eyes." "Stick out your tongue." These are the simplest commands to follow. As you move away from the head and toward the body, the commands become slightly more difficult. "Show me thumbs up" and "wiggle your toes" are good tests of cortical control of the extremities.
- *Middle level of questions/commands:*
  - "Who is the president of the United States?" The family can tell you if the patient should know the answer. You can also ask about current local or global events.
  - "Touch your right ear with your left thumb." Two-step commands require attention and comprehension.
- *Higher level of questions/commands:*
  - "How many quarters are there in $2.25 [$1.50 is easier]?" For patients who are poor at math, ask them to spell their name forward and backward.

Language comprehension deficits may appear as altered mental status. If you get the hunch that your patient is simply not understanding your questions, try to get him to mimic your doing things such as winking, sticking out your tongue, or holding your arms up.

If language comprehension appears largely intact, assess your patient's naming and repetition ability. Point to your pen, cell phone, belt, or watch and ask him to name them. Make a note of your patient's answers because subtle language deficits may be difficult to pick up. For example, if your patients calls the pen "a pencil" or the watch "a clock," there may be a language aphasia. Assess repetition by asking the patient to repeat "no ifs, ands, or buts."

Also note if there is slurred speech. Mild dysarthria may be noticeable by only the family. Moderate dysarthria is when you notice it. Severe dysarthria is when you can hardly understand what the patient is saying.

2. Cranial nerves.

- CN I: Sense of smell can be tested with coffee found at the nurse's station. This nerve is not often checked.

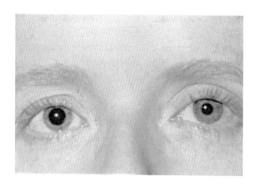

FIGURE 1-4: Example of asymmetric pupil. From Tasman W, Jaeger E. *The Wills Eye Hospital Atlas of Clinical Ophthalmology*, 2nd Ed. Lippincott Williams & Wilkins, 2001.

- CN II: Visual acuity in both eyes can be tested with a Snell pocket vision chart. Check for pupil symmetry and reactivity to light. An example of asymmetric pupils is seen in Figure 1-4.
- CN III, IV, VI: Extraocular movements are assessed by asking the patient to follow your finger right, left, up, down, and to all four corners. Watch the patient's eyes for dysconjugation and ask the patient if he ever sees double as the eyes move around. In Figure 1-5, an exam of eye movements

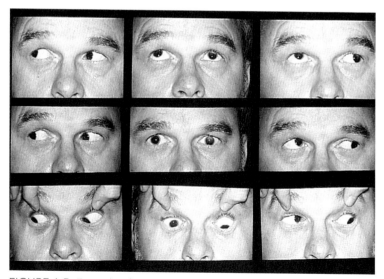

FIGURE 1-5: Example of examination of eye movements in a patient with a right cranial nerve IV lesion. He has incomplete movements of the right eye when looking far to his upper left and lower left.

reveals a cranial nerve IV palsy, especially when the patient looks up to his left and down to his left.

- CN V: Check sensation to soft touch, pinprick, temperature, and vibration in the V1, V2, and V3 distributions of both sides of the face.
- CN VII: Note whether there is a facial droop at rest, then ask the patient to smile to see if the facial muscles appear symmetric. Ask the patient to close his eyes tight and try to pry open his eyelids. Note any asymmetry (Fig. 1-6).
- CN VIII: Check hearing to finger rub or number whispering in both ears.
- CN IX: Note any asymmetry in elevation of the palate when the patient opens his or her mouth wide to say "Ahhhh."
- CN X: Note any voice hoarseness.
- CN XI: Check the strength of the sternocleidomastoid muscles by asking the patient to turn his head all the way to one side and resist your effort to turn the head back.
- CN XII: Note any tongue deviation when the patient sticks out his tongue. Use the patient's teeth as a reference because facial droops can make the tongue appear to deviate.

3. *Motor exam.* Assess for muscle atrophy by observing the muscles in the limbs and face. Make a special note of focal atrophy of muscles. A common place of atrophy includes the intrinsic muscles of the hand.

Note the muscle tone in arms and legs by asking the patient to relax while you shake his or her limbs back and forth. Note any stiffness, spasms, and asymmetry.

FIGURE 1-6: Depiction of complete seventh nerve palsy showing a droopy eyelid, and flattened nasolabial fold. From Moore KL and Agur A. Essential Clinical Anatomy, 2nd Ed. Philadelphia: Lippincott Williams & Wilkins, 2002.

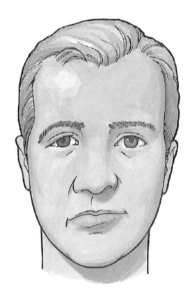

Strength is measured on a subjective 5-point scale:

5 Normal
4 Weaker than usual
3 Can move against gravity
2 Can move, but not against gravity
1 Muscle twitching only
0 No movement

Test the following muscles by asking the patient to maximally flex or extend and resist your pushing back. For each test, use one hand to test the patient's strength and the other hand to stabilize the joint to isolate the muscle.

- Neck flexion: "Touch your chin to your chest and resist me pushing back."
- Neck extension: "Look up, swing your head back, and don't let me push your head back down."
- Shoulder abduction/adduction: "Lift up your elbows at your side and don't let me push up or down."
- Biceps: "Hold your fists to your chest and don't let me pull them out."
- Triceps: "Now bring your fist down to the bed and don't let me push it up."
- Wrist extension: "Hold your wrists back like you're stopping traffic. Don't let me push them down."
- Wrist flexion: "Make a fist, bring your wrists down, and don't let me push them up."
- Finger extension: "Hold your fingers out straight like a board. Don't let me bend them."
- Finger flexion: "Grab my fingers and don't let me open your fist."
- Finger abduction: "Spread your fingers out and don't let me squeeze them in."
- Hip flexion: "Lift your knees up in the air and don't me push them down."
- Hip extension: "Hold your knees down on the bed and don't let me lift them up."
- Knee flexion: "Bend your knees and keep them bent. Don't let me straighten your legs."
- Knee extension: "Straighten your legs and don't let me bend them."
- Ankle dorsiflexion (or ankle extension): "Bring your toes and ankle up toward your head and hold them there. Don't let me push them down."
- Ankle plantar flexion (or ankle flexion): "Push down with your feet like you're pushing on the gas."
- Test for pronator drift by asking the patient to hold out his arms, palms up, fingers spread, and eyes closed. Make note of pronator drift of the hand turning inward, or nonpronator drift of the arm up or down with the palm still facing up.

4. *Sensory exam.* The sensory exam is very subjective and is often inconsistent. Do not spend too much time on the sensory exam unless the chief complaint is sensory in nature.

Briefly compare sensation between the two sides of the body using at least three of the following four modalities: pinprick, soft touch, temperature, and vibration. The best places to check for sensory loss are the hands and the feet. Check for proprioceptive loss by asking the patient to close his eyes while you gently move his large toes up and down.

5. *Reflexes.* While you are on your neurology rotation, put away the Taylor reflex hammer and find a Queen Square hammer.

Check reflexes by placing your fingers over the tendons you will strike and strike the back of your fingers with the reflex hammer. By using this technique, you are sure to transmit the force directly to the tendons and you do not hurt your patient.

The following tendons should be checked for reflexes: bicep, tricep, brachioradialis, patella, and ankle. Superficial reflexes are limited to Babinski's and snout testing.

Reflexes are scored based on a scale of pluses:

- 0 No reflexes
- 1+ Reflex only with reinforcement
- 2+ Normal reflexes
- 3+ Spread of reflexes
- 4+ Clonus

Reinforcement is achieved by asking the patient to bite down or pull apart her clasped hands. *Reflex spread* refers to a movement of a muscle group that is not directly attached to the tendon being tested. For example, if the fingers flex when the bicep tendon is struck, that is considered spread. Clonus is the presence of persistent reflex activity when a joint is struck or extended. For example, if you jerk and hold your patient's ankle in a dorsiflexed position and you can feel the ankle flexing more than once, that is clonus. Make a note of the number of times you feel the ankle flexing in clonus.

6. *Coordination.* The two best tests of coordination are finger-to-nose and heel-to-shin. Ask your patient to use her index finger to touch your finger, which you've placed in front of her. Then ask your patient to touch her nose. Move your finger to different points in front of her and ask her to go back and forth between her nose and your finger. The farther you make the patient stretch to reach your finger, the more likely you will find a subtle deficit. Compare right and left sides.

Cerebellar ataxia is seen when the shaking worsens as the target is neared. Weakness can cause shaking of the hand but it is usually shaking the whole way up and does not worsen as the target nears. Essential tremors can be seen as the patient stretches her arms out and is almost always bilateral.

Ankle-to-shin testing can be difficult for patients who are not flexible. If she can, ask your patient to place her heel on the opposite knee and run her heel up and down the shin. Compare right and left sides.

7. *Gait.* A full gait examination is described in Chapter 7, Gait Disorders and Falls. In brief, ask your patient to stand and walk a few paces in her normal gait. If possible, ask her to walk on her toes and heels and make a note of any difficulties. Ask your patient to walk tandem with one foot in front of the other, as in a sobriety test. You might want to hold on to your patient to make sure she does not fall. Finally, test for a Romberg sign by having your patient stand straight, feet together, with eyes closed. A significant swaying or any falls is considered "positive."

THE PSYCHIATRIC PHYSICAL EXAM—MENTAL STATUS EXAM

The mental status exam (MSE) is the psychiatrist's physical exam. There are 12 components of the MSE that are assessed throughout the interview process. In contrast to the general physical or neurologic physical exams, the MSE does not involve touching the patient. Rather, the MSE is compiled by observation and interview.

The twelve components of the MSE are the following:

1. *Appearance.* Assess the overall physical appearance of your patient. Include chronologic and apparent age, height, weight, manner of dress, and hygiene.
2. *Behavior.* Observe how your patient behaves, sits, gestures, and moves during the interview with special attention paid to the patient's cooperation and interaction with you. Your notes should include tics, tremors, and a slouching posture, if present.
3. *Speech (not language).* The primary components of speech are rate, rhythm, volume, and tone, but also note other features of speech, such as stuttering, mannerisms, accents, as well as loud, emotional, or labored speech.
4. *Mood/affect.* Mood is the emotional state described by the patient. Affect is the outward show of emotion described by you. Affect is described by quality—elevated, euthymic, depressed—as well as by range and stability. When you note your observations, also note whether the patient's affect is appropriate to that particular situation.
5. *Thought*:
   a. *Process.* Is the patient making logical sense? Describe the thought process as pressured, a flight of ideas (quickly jumping from one thought to the next), blocked thoughts, and illogical thinking.
   b. *Content.* Note whether the patient's thinking is logical but crazy in content. A patient may make perfect sense talking about a *delusional* idea. A delusion is a fixed but false belief.
6. *Perceptions.* Note hallucinations (seeing something when nothing is there) and/or illusions (seeing something when something else is there). Ask for details about hallucinations, such as hearing voices, including

what the voices are saying. Specifically ask if the voices are commanding the patient to harm himself or others.

7. *Cognition.* Note a general description of intelligence, concentration, and higher cognitive ability.

8. *Consciousness.* Note the level of consciousness during the interview. Examples include clear, fluctuating, and clouded.

9. *Orientation.* Four areas of orientation are person, place, date, and situation.

10. *Memory.* Testing of short- and long-term memory can be assessed by asking the patient to remember a name and address: John Brown, 42 Market Street, Chicago. Make sure the patient can repeat it (task of attention) and then recall the name and address 5 minutes later. Long-term memory can be assessed by asking about memories from the patient's childhood. For memory and orientation testing, the Mini Mental Status Exam is a short and useful standardized measurement.

11. *Judgment.* This subjective assessment may be difficult to make in a short interview. Comment on whether you believe the patient is able to make sound judgments.

12. *Insight.* Does the patient understand what his problems are? Is he working toward understanding and solving them?

PERFORMING NEUROLOGIC AND PSYCHIATRIC EXAMS

At first, you may find yourself spending a lot of time examining patients on the neurology service. Compared to other clinical services in the hospital, the neurology service still depends on the physical exam for localizing the disease process. Take your time and learn to perform the complete neurologic and psychiatric exams. As you acquire experience on the neurology and psychiatry clerkships, you will be able to tailor your exams to the specific problem.

WHAT YOU NEED TO REMEMBER

- Neurology is a unique speciality of medicine that relies heavily on the history and neurologic exam.
- On first starting the neurology clerkship, you need to learn how to perform the complete neurologic and psychiatric exams.
- Use a one-liner summary to quickly communicate with your residents, attending physician, and other team members.
- By the end of the clerkship, your goal is to be able to perform a problem-specific neurologic exam, reason through the localization of the lesion, and offer a limited differential diagnosis of the disease.

SUGGESTED READINGS

A very useful online resource for medical students to learn how to perform a complete physical exam is the University of Utah Web site: http://library.med.utah.edu/neurologicexam/html/home_exam.html.

This Web site contains videos and descriptions of each component of the exam.

Schwartzman R. *Neurologic Examination*. Hoboken, NJ: Wiley-Blackwell; one edition, 2006, is a heavy volume of very detailed instructions for performing a neurologic exam and is a good reference.

Introduction to Neuroradiology

OVERVIEW

Imaging of the central nervous system (CNS) plays a vital role in the diagnosis of diseases that affect the brain, head, neck, and spinal cord. A general understanding of the imaging techniques used by the neuroradiologist is necessary to understand the care of many patients in the clinical neurosciences. This chapter will introduce fundamental concepts in neuroradiology with a practical bent and should serve medical students as a first primer in understanding the role of the radiologist in the care of patients with pathology of the CNS.

UNDERSTANDING COMPUTED TOMOGRAPHY

Computed tomography (CT) is a cross-sectional imaging technique that uses x-rays, which are a form of ionizing radiation. Information is obtained by passing a thin x-ray beam through the patient from different orientations and measuring the corresponding x-ray attenuation. The data acquired are reconstructed to produce cross-sectional images based on relative x-ray attenuation, measured as Hounsfield units (HU) on a scale from minus to plus infinity. The higher the HU a pixel is assigned, the brighter it appears on CT and vice versa.

Although not technically correct, it is a useful simplification to initially think of denser materials as attenuating more x-rays and vice versa. For example, the calcium in bone will be displayed as brighter compared to brain parenchyma, as opposed to air, which is less dense and therefore darker (see Table 2-1 and Fig. 2-1). In reality, the interactions of x-ray photons with matter at the subatomic level govern attenuation and are only partially the result of density, a phenomenon that we take advantage of in using iodine-containing contrast agents, for instance. The physics of radiology is a complex topic largely beyond the scope of this chapter; radiologists typically study the topic in detail throughout their training.

Because the human eye cannot perceive an infinite number of shades of gray, only a portion of the data is displayed at any given time; the so-called CT window indicates the range of Hounsfield units displayed. In addition, raw data may be passed separately through various processing algorithms to best display soft tissue or bone. Unlike MRI, in which bone is not well visualized, CT can display osseous structures in remarkable detail; the bony structures should be the first place you look if you are uncertain

TABLE 2-1

Relative X-ray Attenuation in Hounsfield Units (HU) of Various Tissues within the Brain (Approximate)

Tissue	Attenuation (HU)
Bone	1,000
Blood	60–100
Grey matter	37
White matter	30
Water	0
Fat	−120
Air	−1,000

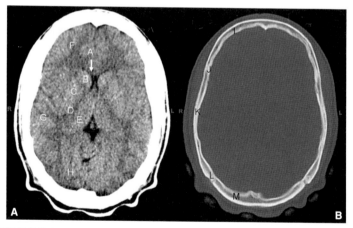

FIGURE 2-1: Normal noncontrast axial CT of the head. Note that air surrounding the head is dark whereas bone is displayed as bright and that the appearance changes depending on what window is applied and whether the bone or soft tissue algorithm was used. **A.** Brain window. *A*, frontal horn, right lateral ventricle; *B*, head of caudate nucleus; *C*, lentiform nucleus (putamen and globus pallidus); *D*, internal capsule, posterior limb; *E*, thalamus; *F*, frontal lobe; *G*, temporal lobe; *H*, occipital lobe. **B.** Bone window. *I*, frontal bone; *J*, coronal suture; *K*, parietal bone; *L*, lambdoid suture; *M*, occipital bone.

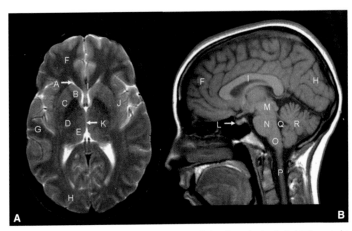

FIGURE 2-2: Normal noncontrast MRI of the head. **A.** Axial T2-weighted image with fat saturation. *A* (*arrow*), frontal horn, right lateral ventricle; *B*, head of caudate nucleus; *C*, lentiform nucleus (putamen and globus pallidus); *D*, internal capsule, posterior limb; *E*, thalamus; *F*, frontal lobe; *G*, temporal lobe; *H*, occipital lobe; *I*, corpus callosum; *J*, insular cortex; *K* (*arrow*), third ventricle. **B.** Sagittal T1-weighted image. Note how the corpus callosum (*I*, a white matter structure) is brighter than the grey matter of the cortex (*F*, *H*). *L* (*arrow*), pituitary gland; *M*, midbrain; *N*, pons; *O*, medulla oblongata; *P*, cervical spinal cord; *Q*, fourth ventricle; *R*, cerebellum.

whether you are looking at a CT scan or an MRI (compare Fig. 2-1B to 2-2A).

CLINICAL PEARL

If you are not sure whether you are looking at a CT or an MRI scan, look for the skull bone. If the skull bone is bright white, it is a CT scan. If the skull bone looks black or absent, it is an MRI.

UNDERSTANDING MAGNETIC RESONANCE IMAGING

Magnetic resonance imaging (MRI, also called MR imaging, or just MR) is a cross-sectional technique that is based on the concentration and relaxation characteristics of hydrogen protons in a strong magnetic field. The primary source of hydrogen in the brain is water, and pathology can often be perceived because of differences in local water content. MRI is extremely sensitive to the detection of disease processes in the brain. For example, MRI is more sensitive than CT in the detection of the early changes of stroke. MRI also has the

TABLE 2-2

Summary of Signal Characteristics of Various Tissues within the Brain

Scan	Uses	CSF	Lesion	Blood	Bone
CT	Acute setting	Dark	Dark	Bright	Bright
T1	Anatomy	Dark	Dark	Varies with age of bleed	Dark
T2	Lesion detection	Bright	Bright	Varies with age of bleed	Dark
FLAIR	Lesion detection	Dark	Bright	Varies with age of bleed	Dark

advantage of multiplanar imaging, as images can be directly obtained in the axial, sagittal, or coronal planes for better definition of anatomy, as opposed to CT, in which sagittal and coronal images can only be indirectly obtained from the axially acquired data set via postprocessing techniques.

Basic MRI pulse sequences for brain include T1-weighted imaging, T2-weighted imaging, fluid-attenuated inversion recovery (FLAIR) imaging, and diffusion-weighted imaging (DWI). Table 2-2 summarizes signal characteristics of various tissues within the brain.

T2-Weighted Imaging

T2-weighted images are primarily used for lesion detection. CSF and fluid are bright, and white matter is darker than grey matter on T2-weighted images (Fig. 2-2a).

T1-Weighted Imaging

T1-weighted images are primarily used to define anatomy. CSF and water are dark, and white matter is brighter than grey matter on T1-weighted images (Fig. 2-2b). Additionally, IV contrast (gadolinium) can be given to visualize the intracranial vessels and to delineate breakdown in the blood-brain barrier (Fig. 2-3).

Fluid-Attenuated Inversion Recovery Imaging

FLAIR images are essentially T2 weighted with a suppressed signal from CSF. As such, CSF is dark, but abnormal fluid is brighter and therefore more conspicuous on FLAIR images (Fig. 2-4).

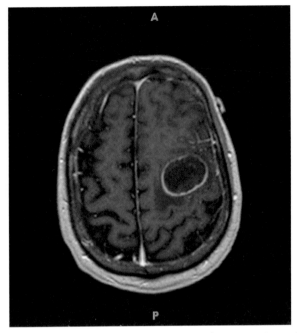

FIGURE 2-3: Example of T1 post–contrast MRI showing a ring enhancing lesion in the left parietal lobe. The ring is created by intravenous gadolinium that leaks across disrupted blood-brain barrier.

Diffusion-Weighted Imaging

Diffusion-weighted imaging (DWI) evaluates the diffusion of water molecules within the brain. Because of failure of the Na/K ATPase on the neuronal cellular membrane, electrolytes (Na and K) and water are trapped in cells and thus are restricted in their diffusion. Such regions appear bright on DWI images within minutes of ischemia onset, and this technique has greatly increased the sensitivity of MRI for detecting early ischemic infarct (Fig. 2-5).

UNDERSTANDING OTHER IMAGING TECHNIQUES

Although medical students will most commonly encounter only CTs and MRIs in the care of their neurologic patients, it is important to know about the various other techniques used by the neuroradiologist.

Fluoroscopy

Fluoroscopy involves the real-time visualization of x-ray or CT images and is used, for instance, by the radiologist in securing access to the subarachnoid space

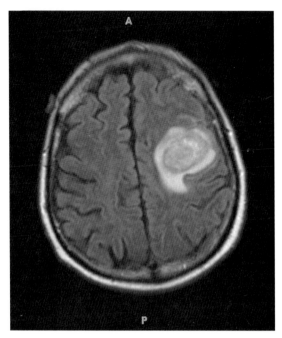

FIGURE 2-4: T2 Flair image of the same lesion from Figure 2.3. Note the hyperintensity surrounding the lesion indicative of edema.

in the spine (if lumbar puncture has been repeatedly unsuccessful at the bedside) or in the image-guided biopsy of lesions of the head and neck or spinal column.

Myelography

Myelography involves direct injection of contrast into the subarachnoid space under fluoroscopy, commonly followed by CT imaging, and allows for excellent visualization of the space surrounding the spine and spinal nerve roots. Myelography is most commonly used in patients who, for whatever reason (such as the presence of a pacemaker that contains copper wires), are unable to undergo MRI of the spine. It is also sometimes used in the preoperative or postoperative setting.

Angiography

Diagnostic catheter angiography involves direct puncture of a peripheral *artery* and the manipulation of a catheter under fluoroscopic guidance within the arterial system for direct injection of contrast into the arteries of the head and neck or spine. This technique has been partially supplanted in its diagnostic capacity at many centers with improvements in CT angiography (CTA) and MR

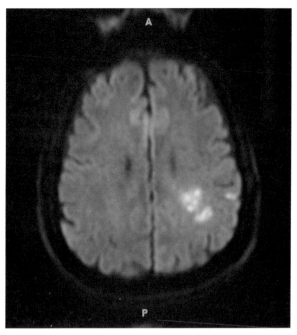

FIGURE 2-5: Example of a diffusion-weighted image of a stroke in the left parietal lobe.

angiography (MRA), which typically require only injection of contrast via a peripheral intra*venous* catheter (CTA) or not at all (MRA, Fig. 2-6), but which may have lesser sensitivity for some pathologies. Neurointerventional radiologists use the techniques of catheter angiography to deploy small coils or inject glue or other agents to percutaneously treat aneurysms, vascular malformations, or tumors among other pathologies. Emergent thrombolysis can also be attempted in certain stroke patients through direct intra-arterial injection of thrombolytic medications. The neurointerventional radiologist can offer percutaneous therapy through a subcentimeter dermotomy for vascular access; there are often substantial benefits to the patient in using this approach instead of open neurosurgical procedures. The trend toward intravascular procedures and away from open surgical procedures has resulted in fewer complications, reduced hospital stays, and more rapid patient recovery.

MR Spectroscopy

MR spectroscopy (MRS) allows for the detection of metabolites in the brain and is used at some centers in the diagnosis of neoplasm and neurodegenerative diseases, for instance.

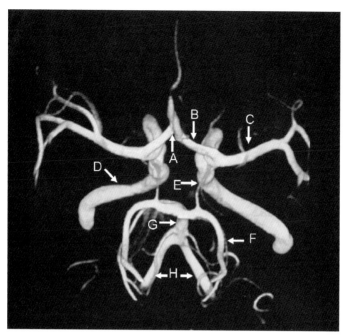

FIGURE 2-6: Magnetic resonance angiography (MRA) of the circle of Willis obtained without intravenous contrast. A, anterior communicating artery; B, anterior cerebral artery; C, middle cerebral artery; D, internal carotid artery; E, posterior communicating artery; F, posterior cerebral artery; G, basilar artery; H, vertebral arteries.

Perfusion Imaging

Perfusion imaging with either CT perfusion (CTP) or MR perfusion (MRP) following the administration of contrast demonstrates time-attenuation (CT) or time-intensity (MRI) curves. It is typically used in assessing the differential perfusion of regions of the brain in suspected neoplasm (increased perfusion) or stroke (decreased perfusion). With regard to ischemic stroke, the region of the brain *unaffected* by cytotoxic edema (restricted diffusion) but that demonstrates decreased perfusion is said to represent the penumbra, or the region at risk of impending infarction.

Plain Film X-rays

Last, plain film x-ray evaluation of the spine is still commonly used in the initial assessment of the spinal column. Plain film radiography of the head has been largely supplanted by CT.

CT OR MRI: WHICH IMAGING STUDY TO ORDER WHEN

The two most widely used brain imaging modalities in teaching hospitals are CT scanning and MRI. They each have their advantages and disadvantages in any particular case and you will need to know when to order a CT scan versus an MRI. Table 2-3 summarizes the advantages and disadvantages of each.

CT

The primary types of CT used are noncontrast CT, contrast-enhanced CT, and CT angiography.

Noncontrast CT

In the acute setting, noncontrast CT is often the preferred first-line imaging modality because it is quick, is easily available, and has few contraindications. It is an appropriate initial scan to order when dealing with trauma, stroke, headache, or changes in mental status to get a quick glimpse into the head. CT is readily available in the emergency room and is a rapid technique for imaging the brain—most exams last only a few seconds. Aside from the risks associated with exposure to ionizing radiation, CT is a safe and effective technique.

The primary disadvantage of CT is that early disease processes may escape detection. For example, ischemic stroke is often not detected within

TABLE 2-3
Advantages and Disadvantages of CT versus MRI

	CT	MRI
Speed	Faster (seconds)	Slower (minutes to hours)
Availability	More available	Often less available
Cost	Lower	Higher
Radiation	Yes	No
Detection hyper-acute infarct	Limited within 6 hours	Excellent within minutes
Trauma	Acute setting	Subacute setting
Bone pathology	Well visualized	Often difficult to visualize
Resolution/contrast	Lower	Higher

the first 6 hours by noncontrast head CT. In fact, if CT detects a stroke, you know the stroke occurred >6 hours previously.

Contrast-Enhanced CT

Contrast-enhanced CT is reserved for imaging brain tumors and infections/abscesses and is used to visualize the intracranial vessels. It usually does not play an important role in the acute setting as contrast can obscure small bleeds. CT contrast is not harmless and requires consideration of three important factors:

1. *Allergy to contrast or iodine.* It is generally best to avoid contrast in patients with allergies, but premedication with steroids can be attempted if the contrast study is very important.
2. *Potential kidney toxicity.* Kidney toxicity by the contrast dye typically takes 2 to 3 days to be evident in the renal function as detected by creatinine clearance. In patients with borderline kidney disease, normal saline should be given before and after contrast to help prevent the toxicity.
3. *Diabetic patients.* Diabetics taking metformin should wait 24 hours after stopping the metformin to get the contrast because the combination may cause severe lactic acidosis in a small percentage of diabetics.

CT Angiography

CT angiography (CTA) differs from typical contrast-enhanced CT in the rate of contrast administration and often in the technical aspects of image acquisition and reconstruction. CTA allows for 3D visualization of the major arterial structures of the head and neck and is commonly used in the assessment of significant stenosis or an aneurysm. It requires significant computer postprocessing of the images.

MRI

MRI uses a strong magnetic field. For patients with certain implanted devices, such as pacemakers, MRI may be contraindicated or relatively contraindicated. The theory is that the strong magnetic field in an MRI machine creates a current in the conductive material that passes through the field. In the copper lead of a pacemaker, for example, the beating motion of the heart in the MR magnetic field creates a small current that heats the copper by 1° Celsius. That increase in temperature may displace the lead from the precise location where it is implanted in the heart tissue.

MRI exams typically last 20 minutes to 1 hour, depending on which pulse sequences are performed, and are therefore more physically demanding on the patient (and require the patient to stay still and lie flat throughout the duration of the exam). The MR machine creates a loud, pounding noise that can be annoying, even with earplugs. Some patients may require sedation for the exam to obtain diagnostically adequate images, especially children and claustrophobic patients.

MRI is more sensitive to the presence of small amounts of blood and edema than conventional CT scans, which makes it a very useful modality in the subacute setting once a patient has been stabilized. MRI with contrast is useful for further characterizing known or suspected mass lesions or in detecting small lesions that might be missed on CT.

Brain MRI with Diffusion-Weighted Imaging

Brain MRI with diffusion-weighted imaging (DWI) can detect the early changes of stroke within minutes, whereas detectable attenuation differences on CT may not be seen until >6 hours after the stroke.

Contrast-Enhanced Studies in MRI

Contrast-enhanced studies in MRI require assessment of renal function. Patients with renal dysfunction may be at risk of nephrogenic systemic fibrosis (NSF), a rare but serious and sometimes fatal complication in which gadolinium contrast material deposits in the skin and induces a serious fibrotic reaction. The contrast administered for MRI is different from that administered for CT. A history of an allergic reaction to contrast on CT does not necessarily preclude the administration of contrast on MRI or vice versa.

MR Angiography

MR angiography (MRA) allows for 3D visualization of the major arterial structures of the head and neck and, similar to CTA, may be used in assessing patients for vascular stenosis or an aneurysm. MR venography (MRV) is commonly used to assess patency of the major venous structures of the head. Unlike CTA, both MRA and MRV may be performed without intravenous contrast in patients with altered renal function.

COMMON SIGNIFICANT PATHOLOGIC FINDINGS

There are a few significant pathologic findings seen on CT/MRI that medical students should be able to identify. These common significant pathologic findings include hemorrhage, epidural hematomas, subdural hematomas, subarachnoid hemorrhage, intraparenchymal/intra-axial hemorrhage, stroke, and transient ischemic attack.

Hemorrhage

Most cases of acute intracranial hemorrhage are caused by trauma, with hypertensive hemorrhages and aneurysms being less common. Hemorrhage is almost always high attenuation in the acute setting on noncontrast CT and is always abnormal in the brain. Hemorrhage can be categorized by location (i.e., intra-axial versus extra-axial). Extra-axial hemorrhage can occur in the

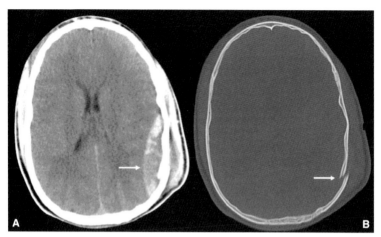

FIGURE 2-7: Axial noncontrast CT of the head with brain (**A**) and bone (**B**) algorithm/ window images demonstrates an epidural hematoma (*arrow*, **A**) centered over the left parietal lobe. Note the typical biconvex shape, associated depressed skull fracture (*arrow*, **B**) and partial decompression into the soft tissues of the left scalp. Epidural hematomas may abut but will not cross sutural lines. Subdural hematomas do not respect suture lines.

epidural, subdural, and subarachnoid spaces. Intra-axial is within the brain or ventricular system.

Epidural Hematomas

Epidural hematomas (Fig. 2-7) typically occur in association with fractures of the temporal bone that cause laceration of the middle meningeal artery. This results in extravasated arterial blood under high pressure, which dissects between the inner table of the skull and the closely applied outer layer of the dura mater. Epidural hematomas do not cross sutures and have a characteristic biconvex or lentiform shape. Because epidural hematomas imply an arterial source, they can rapidly lead to accumulation of blood and increased intracranial pressure, which can result in rapid brain herniation and death. The classic clinical scenario is blunt trauma severe enough to cause an immediate but temporary loss of consciousness followed by a lucid interval of minutes to a few hours, followed by subsequent rapid deterioration. Epidural hematomas are a neurosurgical emergency and must be surgically drained as soon as possible.

Subdural Hematomas

Subdural hematomas (Fig. 2-8) are usually secondary to disruption of the bridging veins between the cerebral cortex and the dural sinuses. Acutely,

FIGURE 2-8: Axial non-contrast CT of the head demonstrates bilateral subdural hematomas with relatively hyperattenuating blood products layering posteriorly in a dependent position (*solid arrows*) and less attenuating blood products anteriorly (*dashed arrows*). Note that the collections traverse both coronal sutures but do not enter the sulci, helpful distinguishing characteristic of subdural hematomas from epidural and subarachnoid blood products, respectively.

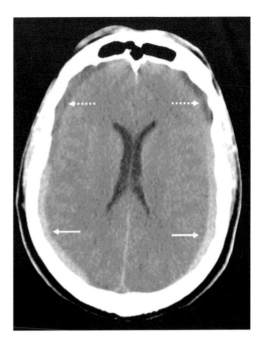

CT will show a crescentic high-attenuation rim of blood between the skull and gray matter, often with mass effect on the ipsilateral ventricular system. Subdural hematomas can spread along the cerebral convexities, freely crossing sutures and appearing thin on axial sections, but, in fact, they represent a large volume of blood. Confined by dural structures such as the tentorium and falx, subdural hematomas do not cross the midline.

Subarachnoid Hemorrhage

Subarachnoid hemorrhage (Fig. 2-9A) is most commonly caused by trauma or aneurysm (Fig. 2-9B). It is usually seen acutely as a hyperdensity that conforms to the cortical sulci and gyri or that collects in the basilar cisterns. Patients can present with an abrupt onset of headache ("thunderclap headache" or "worst headache of my life"), meningeal signs, and sometimes a decreased level of consciousness or coma. The most common causes of atraumatic subarachnoid hemorrhage are berry aneurysms, which usually occur at the bifurcations of major intracranial arteries near the circle of Willis. Similar to traumatic subarachnoid hemorrhage, subarachnoid hemorrhage from berry aneurysms fills the basal cisterns with high-density blood on CT.

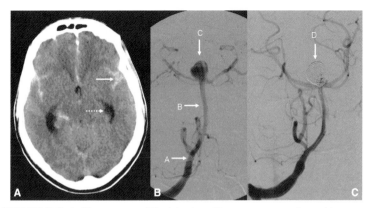

FIGURE 2-9: **A.** Noncontrast CT of the head in a man presenting with severe headache demonstrates diffuse hemorrhage, for instance, in the sylvian fissure on the left (*solid arrow*). Blood products were also noted to fill the basal cisterns and prominently extend into sulci overlying both cerebral hemispheres, characteristics of subarachnoid hemorrhage. There is hydrocephalus as a result of intracranial hemorrhage with dilatation of the lateral ventricles (*dashed arrow*). **B.** On catheter angiography with injection of the right vertebral artery (*A*) contrast fills the basilar artery (*B*) as well as its branches with a large aneurysm of the basilar tip (*C*). **C.** The postprocedural result after the interventional neuroradiologist has percutaneously placed coils (*D*) within the aneurysm, effectively excluding blood flow.

Intraparenchymal/Intra-Axial Hemorrhage

Intraparenchymal/intra-axial hemorrhage (Fig. 2-10) can be seen in the setting of trauma, tumors, vascular malformations, hypertension, amyloid angiopathy, or infarction. Intraparenchymal hemorrhage caused by traumatic injury is usually seen within the region of contusions and petechial hemorrhages in the brain periphery. Penetrating trauma usually causes hemorrhage along the path of injury. Hypertensive hemorrhage occurs most frequently in the deep grey matter structures of the brain, such as the basal ganglia or the thalami. The extent of hemorrhage observed on CT belies actual damage to the brain tissue underneath. When the blood clears, repeat imaging will usually show a smaller area of damage within the old hemorrhage. Depending on the location and size, intraparenchymal hemorrhage may be a neurosurgical emergency because of the danger of rapid compression of vital structures and potential mortality in the acute setting.

Stroke and Transient Ischemic Attack

Stroke (Fig. 2-11) and transient ischemic attack (TIA) are both defined as a sudden, severe, focal loss of brain function caused by ischemia. If

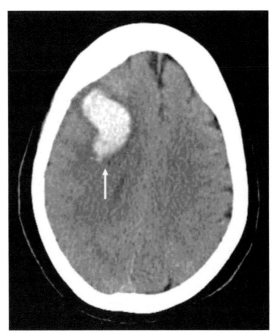

FIGURE 2-10: Acute intraparenchymal hematoma within the high right frontal lobe demonstrating the typical hyperdense appearance with minimal surrounding edema.

symptoms resolve within 24 hours, a transient ischemic attack has occurred. If the symptoms persist for more than 24 hours, the attack is termed a stroke.

CLINICAL PEARL

If MRI shows an area of DWI hyperintensity despite clinical resolution within 24 hours, it is considered a stroke. Thus, MRI diagnosis overrides the clinical diagnosis in this case.

A noncontrast head CT is often still the initial imaging study of choice to exclude hemorrhage, tumor, or other structural lesions that can present with symptoms similar to stroke. It is important to note that TIA and stroke are

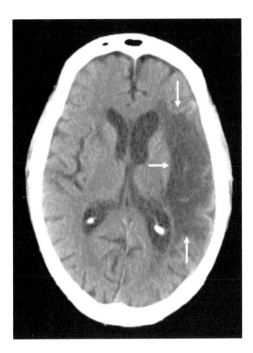

FIGURE 2-11: Noncontrast head CT demonstrates a moderately sized region of hypoattenuation within the arterial distribution of branches of the left middle cerebral artery caused by infarction.

clinical and not radiologic diagnoses, but even when the clinical diagnosis of stroke has already been made, a positive CT or MR exam can still be valuable to clarify the extent and the mechanism of the infarction. However, a negative initial noncontrast CT, especially during the first 6 hours after symptom onset, does not exclude stroke, and small lesions may fail to become apparent for up to 48 to 72 hours or may escape detection altogether. In contrast, MRI with diffusion-weighted imaging is exquisitely sensitive to ischemic injury, even within minutes of symptom onset, and perfusion imaging on MRI or CT can demonstrate areas of hypoperfusion prior to infarction. An MRA or CTA of the circle of Willis and the neck vessels is often performed at the same time to clarify vascular stenosis or sites of occlusion.

TRAINING IN NEURORADIOLOGY

Training in neuroradiology entails 1 year of internship and 4 years of general diagnostic radiology, followed by 1 to 2 years of a neuroradiology fellowship. Additional further years of subspecialized training are possible, such as angiography/neurointervention, head and neck radiology, and pediatric neuroradiology.

WHAT YOU NEED TO REMEMBER

- Neuroradioradiology is an essential adjunct to the practice of neurology and neurosurgery, allowing for highly accurate localization of disease processes and often providing the appropriate diagnosis or significantly narrowing the differential diagnosis established clinically.
- Technologic advances have allowed for capabilities for assessing the central nervous system noninvasively.
- CT and MRI are the mainstays of neuroradiologic practice.
- Diagnostic and interventional neuroradiologists are also able to perform minimally invasive procedures for diagnosis and treatment, often with significant benefits to the patient.

SUGGESTED READINGS

The American Society of Neuroradiology, http://www.asnr.org

Cwinn AA, Grahovac SZ. *Emergency CT Scans of the Head: A Practical Atlas*. St. Louis, MO: Mosby, 1998.

Gillespie JE, Jackson A. *MRI and CT of the Brain*. London, UK: Arnold Publishers, 2000.

Grossman RI, Yousem DM. *Neuroradiology: The Requisites*. St. Louis, MO: Mosby, 2003.

Novelline RA. *Squire's Fundamentals of Radiology*. Cambridge, MA: Harvard University Press, 2004.

Altered Mental Status

THE PATIENT ENCOUNTER

A 69-year-old woman with early dementia was brought in to the emergency department by her son. He says that last night she was complaining of mild headache, fatigue, and subjective fevers. He also says that he heard her get up at least four times last night to use the bathroom. This morning, when he found her in bed, she was difficult to arouse, did not answer his questions, and was too weak to stand. The emergency department physician confirms that she has never had an episode of altered mental status before and calls for a neurology consult.

OVERVIEW

Definition and Pathophysiology

Altered mental status (AMS) is a state of consciousness that is different from baseline. Because there is no nucleus in the brain responsible for consciousness, focal lesions in the brain do not classically cause altered mental status. Rather, consciousness is created by a diffuse network within the cerebral cortex that is dependent on the brainstem to keep it awake (Fig. 3-1). Compromise of consciousness requires either a diffuse metabolic process involving both cerebral cortices or a focal lesion impinging on the reticular activating system in the midbrain.

Epidemiology

The capacity of the brain to buffer itself against diffuse metabolic insults is called *neurologic reserve* and is poorest in the very young (<1 year), the old (>70 years), and the chronically ill. A person of any age can develop altered mental status if the insult overcomes the neurologic reserve. For example, a systemic infection such as pneumonia will not likely cause altered mental status in a 22-year-old medical student with no past medical history. However, if the student develops fulminant rabies encephalitis, even a 22-year-old's mental status will be compromised. In contrast, the brain of an 85-year-old woman with chronic obstructive pulmonary disease (COPD) may not be able to maintain normal consciousness during a simple urinary tract infection because of a poorer neurologic reserve.

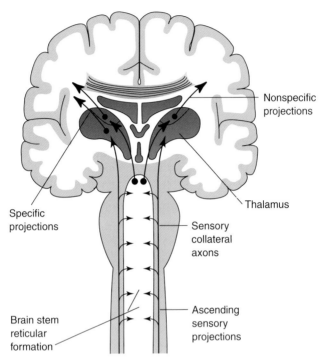

FIGURE 3-1: **The Reticular Activating System (RAS).** The RAS is a diffuse network of nuclei around the cerebral aqueduct in the brainstem that innervates all parts of the cortex via serotonergic and cholinergic projections. The RAS is critical to setting the alertness level of the brain and without innervations by the RAS, the cortex would fall into a comatose state.

ACUTE MANAGEMENT AND WORKUP

Your four-step approach to a patient with altered mental status is the following:

Use the first 15 minutes to ensure that your patient is stable.

When stable, take time to get a complete history, perform a thorough physical examination, and obtain or send off all necessary ancillary testing.

Formulate an assessment that involves localizing the lesion and developing a differential diagnosis.

Discuss the case with your neurology team and develop a treatment plan.

The First 15 Minutes

The goal of the first 15 minutes in evaluating a patient with altered mental status is making sure the patient is stable. When your patient first arrives, you have to get a sense about whether she is getting worse, is getting better, or is stably altered. In someone you have never met who is most likely unable to communicate with you, this is a very difficult task! Therefore, for at least the first 15 minutes, do not leave your altered patient unattended.

Initial Assessment

As always, your first assessment should be the ABCs: airway, breathing, and circulation. The very next thing you must do is to determine if this patient is at risk for impending harm. In other words, is this patient going to die in the next few minutes if you do not intervene? Follow these quick steps in first evaluating any new patient with an altered mental status:

1. *Check the patient's vital signs.* Make sure the patient's blood pressure and pulse are high enough to perfuse the brain, and make sure the oxygen saturation is at baseline or higher.
2. *Find out how quickly the patient's mental status is declining.* For this step, you need to gather information from a reliable source such as a physician, nurse, or family member who has been with the patient. *If the mental status is declining over a matter of minutes, get help!* Do not start your workup until you are sure your patient is hemodynamically stable and will be alive by the end of your workup!
3. *Look for obvious emergent signs that require rapid attention*:
   • Seizure activity
   • Asymmetric dilated unreactive pupils or symmetric pinpoint pupils (Fig. 3-2).

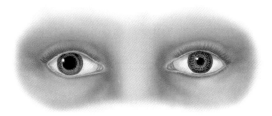

FIGURE 3-2: **Pupils.** An asymmetric dilated pupil (>1 mm more dilated than the other pupil), is consistent with brainstem herniation and is a life-threatening condition that will lead to death within minutes if not reversed. Symmetric pinpoint pupils are usually due to narcotic overdose but can also reflect damage to pons. From Bickley, LS and Szilagyi, P. *Bates' Guide to Physical Examination and History Taking*, 8th Ed. Philadelphia: Lippincott Williams & Wilkins, 2003.

- Hemiparesis/neglect as seen when the patient totally ignores everything on the left side of her world, including you, until you move to the right side of her world.
- Blood sugar less than 60 mg/dL

When you feel comfortable that your patient is stable, take a deep breath and begin the workup.

Admission Criteria and Level of Care Criteria

All patients with acute and persistent altered mental status should be admitted for workup and treatment. If the most likely causes are neurologic, your patient should be admitted to the general neurology service. If there is high suspicion for a medical or surgical cause of altered mental status, your patient might be better served on a primary medicine or surgery service with a neurology consultation.

Patients with altered mental status need to be closely observed at all times because, until the cause is determined, you do not know how much worse your patient is going to get. Make sure there is a nurse or physician nearby who can help you handle your patient if her mental status deteriorates.

When your patient is being transferred to your neurology floor, make sure the nurses on your floor are informed. Tell the accepting nurse what happened with your patient and what the initial workup will be. Ask her to page you if your patient's mental status changes.

If your patient's mental status puts her at risk of harming herself or others, it would be wise to order either restraints or a sitter who can watch your patient.

Restraints come in two varieties: physical (Fig. 3-3) and chemical (sedating medications). Physical restraints can be wrapped around the wrists and

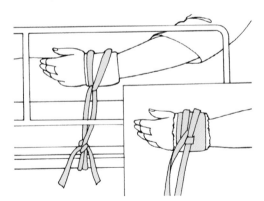

FIGURE 3-3: **Physical restraints.** Physical restraints are designed to keep the patient's arms and legs out of harm's way without causing too much discomfort. From *Nursing Procedures*, 4th Edition. Ambler: Lippincott Williams & Wilkins, 2004.

ankles or around the chest. Physical restraints are not comfortable, so before ordering them, make sure they are in your patient's best interest. Chemical restraints are sedatives and/or antipsychotics. These drugs may keep your patient comfortable while the workup is being performed. Keep in mind that your neurologic exam will become clouded by these drugs and that these drugs have many neurologic side effects that you must consider before ordering. As soon as your patient recovers to the point that restraints are no longer needed, please have them removed as soon as possible.

The First 24 Hours

In patients with altered mental status, the history often provides the most important clues to the cause. Unfortunately, the patient is often too altered to provide you with that important information. Interview the patient's family to compile your history.

History

Your goals in evaluating a patient with AMS are the following:

1. *Determine the baseline mental status of the patient and how altered it is.* This is best obtained from family, friends, witnesses, and previous physicians who know your patient—do not hesitate to call people. Individuals with little neurologic reserve (e.g., a person with severe Alzheimer disease) are brittle and become altered from any metabolic perturbation such as an infection or medication overuse. In contrast, patients who are very high functioning with careers and who take care of many people in addition to themselves do not easily slip down the spectrum to become altered and should prompt concern for a very serious illness.

   Examples of how to broach the topic as well as questions to ask the family include the following: "I would like to get a sense of what your mother was like before she became sick. Is she normally able to handle her daily activities without assistance? Was she handling her own checkbook? Driving to her appointments? Cooking her own meals? Doing her own laundry and dressing herself?"

CLINICAL PEARL

The first things that are lost when an individual's neurologic reserve begins deteriorating are driving and managing finances because these activities take a lot of brain power to do correctly.

---

2. *Identify the acuity of onset.* You want to know how fast the change in mental status occurred. Acuity will help you narrow down your differential

diagnosis. Try to fit the answers down to one of the following six choices:

- Suddenly, over seconds
- Over a few minutes
- Over a few hours
- Over a day or two
- Over the past couple of weeks
- Over the past few months

The acuity of onset and duration of alteration will help narrow down your differential (see the Assessment section later in this chapter).

3. *Determine what type of AMS the patient has.* States of consciousness range from normal to comatose and include normal, lethargic (sleeping but arousable), obtunded (deep sleep and difficult to arouse), and comatose. The term *delirium* is reserved to describe an altered state of consciousness that is waxing and waning, acute in onset, and largely reversible.

4. *Identify any symptoms associated with AMS that the patient experienced prior to the onset of AMS.* Important complaints include headache, fevers, chills (think: meningitis), urinary urgency, frequency, and burning (think: urinary tract infection [UTI]), lightheadedness or dizziness (think: dehydration, arrhythmia, myocardial infarction [MI]), shortness of breath (think: arrhythmia, pulmonary embolism [PE], MI), focal neurologic deficits such as weakness on one side of the body (think: stroke).

5. *Find out if the patient is taking any new medications or has had any recent changes in medication doses.* Be sure you create an accurate list of current medications and ask the family if any new medications have been started or if any of the doses have changed recently. It is also important to know who manages your patient's medications (the patient vs. a family member). Common medications that lead to AMS include antipsychotics (e.g., Haldol), benzodiazepines (e.g., Valium), opiates (e.g., OxyContin), hypoglycemics (e.g., insulin), sleep medications, dopaminergic medications commonly used for restless leg syndrome, and anticholinergics (e.g., Benadryl).

6. *Obtain the patient's past medical history.* In the write-up, note the complete history, but also make special note of previous episodes of altered mental status, immunosuppression by drugs (e.g., steroids) or disease (e.g., HIV), cerebrovascular and/or coronary artery disease, seizures, diabetes, and glucose-lowering therapy.

7. *Obtain the patient's social history.* Understand your patient's living conditions. A patient living alone with dementia should make you suspect dehydration and nutritional deficiencies that can be easily treated. The use of alcohol, as well as prescription and illicit drugs is important to rule out. Be sure to ask the patient and family in a nonjudgmental fashion.

Physical Examination

Perform a complete general and neurologic exam. Refer to Chapter 1, Localization and the Neurologic Exam, for details on the neurologic exam and to Chapter 12, Mood Disorders, for details on the mental status exam.

Make sure to perform the following key parts of the exam:

- *Vital signs.* A low blood pressure or pulse rate may cause insufficient cerebral perfusion, leading to altered mental status; a high temperature may indicate an infection, a drug reaction, or toxicity.
- *Head, eye, ear, nose, and throat (HEENT).* Determine if there is any evidence of trauma from a fall, or a bitten tongue from a seizure.
- *Neck.* Gently move your patient's neck around to see if it is stiff from meningitis or a subarachnoid hemorrhage.
- *Chest.* Is your patient breathing? Make sure you hear good airflow.
- *Neurologic status.* Establish the following:
  - How impaired is the patient's mental status from baseline?
  - Describe how the patient responds to you (if at all).
  - Try to perform as complete a neurologic exam as possible, examining the following:
    - Cranial nerves. Even if your patient is not very cooperative, you can still check a few of the cranial nerves, including pupillary reaction. If your patient will not follow your finger, observe extraocular movements by getting her to look toward a sound on her right and left sides. Alternatively, if you place a mirror in front of her eyes, she may track the reflection with her eyes; check for corneal reflex; observe facial symmetry.
    - Motor response. If your patient cannot cooperate with a motor exam, observe for spontaneous movements. Are they asymmetric? Check the tone in the patient's muscles and try to pinch the limbs to see if they have good strength on withdrawal.
    - Sensory response. Without cooperation, the only sensory test you can perform is response to pain. Start with a gentle pinch and look for a withdrawal response and make a special note of asymmetry.
    - Reflexes. Make sure reflexes and Babinski responses are symmetric.

Labs and Tests to Consider

Consider each lab test carefully instead of indiscriminately checking off every box on the lab draw form.

CLINICAL PEARL

Remember that labs should only confirm what you already suspect. If you're surprised by an abnormal lab value, review the patient's history or physical exam notes to make sure you did not miss anything important!

Key Diagnostic Labs and Tests

The workup for altered mental status is broad and includes neurologic and non-neurologic testing (Table 3-1). Every patient with altered mental status gets a complete blood count and metabolic panel because these tests are sensitive in detecting common non-neurologic systemic causes of mental status such as infection, hypoglycemia, and renal failure.

Imaging and Ancillary Testing

Imaging is critical in localizing the cause of AMS to the brain (Table 3-2). Although a normal CT or MRI of the brain does not rule out a neurologic cause, a visible lesion in the brain should always prompt a thorough neurologic workup.

Assessment

The assessment should comprise three key parts:

- *A succinct, summary sentence that includes the most important aspects of the history, physical, and tests.* For example: "69-year-old woman with an unknown medical history who presents with acute change in mental status, fever, and a stiff neck."
- *Localization.* **In the case of altered mental status, the cerebral cortex is always involved unless there is a focal midbrain lesion compromising the reticular activating system.** Use clues from the history, the physical exam, and imaging to try to tease out other lesions.
- *Differential diagnosis.* The differential diagnosis for altered mental status can be broken down into the following eight categories:
  - *Vascular.* Stroke, TIA, intraparenchymal hemorrhage, subacrachnoid hemorrhage, subdural hematoma, and global cerebral perfusion insufficiency
  - *Infectious.* Meningitis, encephalitis, urinary tract infections, pneumonia, and Creutzfeldt-Jacob disease (rare)
  - *Metabolic.* Dehydration, hypoxia, uremia secondary to acute renal failure, acidemia, hematologic crises such as thrombotic thrombocytopenic purpura (TTP), medication toxicity, alcohol withdrawal and Wernicke-Korsakoff encephalopathy
  - *Inflammatory.* Cerebritis, acute demyelinating encephalomyelitis, sarcoidosis, and central nervous system (CNS) vasculitis
  - *Neoplastic.* Metastatic cancer, primary CNS cancer, paraneoplastic process, and carcinomatous meningitis
  - *Trauma.* Diffuse axonal injury
  - *Allergic.* Adverse reaction to drugs such as benzodiazepines, anticholinergics, and antiemetics
  - *Seizure related.* Status epilepticus, postictal state

TABLE 3-1
Key Laboratory Tests and Rationales for Testing

Test	Rationale
CBC (Complete blood count) with differential	Rule out (r/o) leukocytosis
Basic metabolic panel	R/o evidence of metabolic dysfunction such as acute renal failure (ARF)/uremia, electrolyte imbalance such as hyponatremia
Specific drug levels	E.g. phenytoin, lithium
Ethanol	R/o alcohol intoxication
Urine toxicity	R/o toxic ingestion
Urinalysis	R/o UTI
Blood/urine cultures	If infection is suspected
Lumbar puncture Tube 1: cell count + differential (1.5 mL). Look for WBC to indicate infection/inflammation and RBC for blood in the CNS. Sometimes elevated RBC in the first tube suggests a traumatic spinal tap procedure. Compare to the counts in tube 4.	Indicated if: • CT scan shows no new intracranial abnormalities **and** • There is a fever and/or stiff neck **or** • Known history of aneurysm (to rule out subarachnoid hemorrhage from an aneurysm rupture) **or**

(continued)

TABLE 3-1
Key Laboratory Tests and Rationales for Testing (Continued)

Test	Rationale
Tube 2: glucose, protein (1.5 mL). Low glucose and high protein is suggestive of active infection/inflammatory process.	• The patient is immunosuppressed from medications or illness **or** • MRI shows enhancement of the meninges **or** • There is no other known cause for the altered mental status.

Tube 3: Gram's stain, culture, viral PCRs such as herpes simplex virus and varicella virus, VDRL to rule out neurosyphilis (6 mL).

Tube 4: cell count + differential (1.5 mL). If the WBC is close to the count in tube 1, the value should be considered accurate. Similarly, if the RBC is close to the count in tube 1, you must assume there is blood in the CNS and not simply that the spinaltap was traumatic.

Tube 5: if collected: flow cytometry and cytopathology to rule out malignancy and lymphoma in the appropriate clinical context (8–10 mL).

R/o, Rule out; WBC, white blood cells; RBC, red blood cells; PCRs, polymerase chain reactions, VDRL, Venereal Disease Research Laboratories [test].

TABLE 3-2
Key Imaging Tests and Rationales for Testing

Test	Rationale
Chest x-ray (CXR)	R/o pneumonia
Noncontrast head computed tomography (CT)	R/o intracranial hemorrhage from stroke or subarachnoid hemorrhage, subdural hemorrhage from trauma, previous strokes, and hydrocephalus.
Magnetic resonance imaging (MRI) of head When possible, an MRI is the ideal imaging modality because of the quality of the images and the increased sensitivity to evaluate for stroke, small tumors, and inflammatory neurologic diseases. However, the downsides of MRI are that it takes a long time to perform (up to 1 hour depending on the type of MRI), there are usually long lines in the hospital so it takes hours before your patient is scanned, MRIs of the brain are expensive compared to CT scans ($1,500–$2,400), patients with pacemakers cannot get MRIs, and patients who are claustrophobic may not tolerate lying in the MRI scanner.	Discriminate normal brain from pathology.
Electroencephalogram (EEG)	Evaluate for spikes or sharp waves (seizure activity) or diffuse cerebral slowing (AMS).

The causes of AMS that are based on the duration of the mental status alteration can be found in Table 3-3. Table 3-4 provides a listing of AMS causes that are based on patient age groups.

Treatment

The treatment of altered mental status obviously depends on the cause. Until the cause is determined, all patients should receive the following basic treatments:

1. Stabilization and observation of vital signs, including blood pressure, pulse, and respiratory status
2. Correction of fluid status and nutrition
3. Cessation of any medications that may further alter the mental status
4. Continuation of any home medications that may improve mental status, such as antiepileptics
5. Empiric thiamine, folate, a multivitamin for alcohol withdrawal, and antibiotics for infection (e.g., meningitis), as indicated

Etiology-specific therapy for each of the eight categories in the previous Assessment section is the goal of care once the workup suggests a cause.

EXTENDED INHOSPITAL MANAGEMENT

In general, treatment leads to rapidly improved mental status (<24 hours) if the causes include dehydration, nonneurologic infection, medication toxicity, and/or a postictal state. In cases of persistent altered mental status (>24 hours), more sophisticated testing should be ordered (e.g., an MRI, an electroencephalogram [EEG], and lumbar puncture), depending on the suspected cause.

DISPOSITION

Discharge Goals

Discharge goals are the following:

- Improvement of the mental status back to baseline prior to hospitalization, or, a maximized improvement to a new baseline.
- Explaining to the patient and his or her family what caused the change in the patient's mental status and what was done to reverse it. If possible, teach the patient and his or her family or caretakers how to prevent the situation from occurring again. For example, if the cause is determined to be seizures secondary to poor medication compliance, encourage your patient to take her medication as prescribed.

Outpatient Care

All patients discharged with altered mental status need follow-up after discharge, which should be arranged *before* the patient leaves the hospital. If the

TABLE 3-3

Causes of AMS Based on the Duration of the Alteration

Transient Changes (<1 hour)		Persistent Changes (>1 hour)	
Neurologic	Nonneurologic	Neurologic	Nonneurologic
Seizures	Dehydration	Infection (meningitis/ encephalitis)	Dehydration
Cerebrovascular disease	Hypoglycemia	Cerebrovascular disease	Hypoglycemia
Migraine	Hypoxia/hypercapnia	Seizures, postictal states	Hypoxia/hypercapnia
Syncope	Syncope	Rheumatologic diseases (lupus cerebritis)	Medication/drug/ alcohol toxicity
Trauma	Medication/drug/ alcohol toxicity	Trauma	Nonneurologic infection
	Infection	Liver or kidney disease Medication toxicity	

TABLE 3-4
Causes of AMS Based on Patient Age Groups

Patient Ages Younger than 40 Years		Patient Ages Older than 60 Years	
Neurologic	**Nonneurologic**	**Neurologic**	**Nonneurologic**
Seizures, postictal states	Medication/drug/alcohol toxicity	Seizures, postictal states	Dehydration
Trauma	Infection	Cerebrovascular disease	Systemic infections such as pneumonia or urinary tract infections
Syncope	Syncope	Rheumatologic diseases (lupus cerebritis)	Medication/drug/alcohol toxicity
Migraine		Trauma	Hypoxia/hypercapnia
		Liver or kidney disease	Hypoglycemia

cause was determined to be primarily neurologic, such as seizures, follow-up should be arranged with a neurologist. If the cause was determined to be primarily medical, such as a urinary tract infection, follow-up should be arranged with the patient's primary care physician.

WHAT YOU NEED TO REMEMBER

- Altered mental status is a negative change in mental status from baseline that can range from normal to comatose.
- Neurologic reserve is the buffering ability of the brain. Patients with poor neurologic reserve can easily develop an altered mental status in the setting of even minor systemic metabolic abnormalities.

- In the first 15 minutes, assess the rate of decline in the patient's mental status. If it's rapidly declining, get help immediately.
- The history of the present illness is the key to determining the cause of altered mental status. Find a family member who can answer your questions.
- The physical exam may be limited by your patient's cooperation.
- Workup for altered mental status includes imaging of the head (CT or MRI), blood tests to look for infectious or metabolic abnormalities, and lumbar puncture and/or EEG in the appropriate context.
- Treatment for altered mental status depends on the cause.
- Remember that the most common non-neurologic causes of altered mental status in the elderly are the following: dehydration, urinary tract infection, and medication toxicity.

SUGGESTED READINGS

Brazis PW, Masdeau JC, Biller J. *Localization in Clinical Neurology.* 6th Ed. Philadelphia: Lippincott Williams & Wilkins, 2006.

Flaherty AW, Rost NS. *The Massachusetts General Hospital Handbook of Neurology.* 2nd Ed. Philadelphia: Lippincott Williams & Wilkins, 2007.

Greenberg D, Aminoff MJ, Simon RP. *Clinical Neurology.* 5th Ed. New York: McGraw-Hill/Appleton & Lange, 2002.

Patten JP. *Neurological Differential Diagnosis.* 2nd Ed. New York: Springer, 1998.

4

Weakness

A 64-year-old retired postman presents to the emergency room with weakness of his left arm. He was holding a cup of coffee this morning when suddenly he was unable to hold the cup and spilled the coffee on the floor. Since that time, he says that his left arm feels heavy and he has a hard time controlling it. He has no other complaints at this time. Neurology was consulted.

OVERVIEW

Definition and Pathophysiology

Weakness is one of the more common chief complaints for which a neurologist will be consulted in an emergency room. There are two presentations of weakness: focal and generalized. Focal weakness is the loss of power in a limb (or limbs) or the face while the other parts of the body are unaffected. Generalized weakness is the loss of power of most or all muscles and portends a very different workup and treatment plan.

Recall that movement is a complex process, coordinated by the brain, that involves the central nervous system, the peripheral nervous system, muscles, ligaments, and bones. Weakness can be caused by a problem in any of these areas.

Within the central nervous system, the process of movement takes the following route:

- Movement begins with thought; a thought of movement is conjured by your consciousness.
- Secondarily, the supplemental motor cortical neurons trigger the motor cortex to initiate a movement. The motor neurons in the motor cortex send an impulse down to the appropriate spinal motor neurons, which relay the signal out of the central nervous system into the peripheral nervous system and then synapses at the neuromuscular junction.
- The electrical signal is then converted to a chemical signal that diffuses across the neuromuscular junction to trigger depolarization of the muscle. While the muscle is contracting, a separate inhibitory signal reaches the spinal motor neurons that control the antagonizing muscle. For example, while your biceps contract, your triceps relax.

Let us consider dysfunction at each level of the neuroaxis, starting in the motor cortex. The motor cortex is located on the posterior end of the frontal lobe stretching from the sagittal sinus to the temporal fissure in the pattern of a homunculus (Fig. 4-1). A lesion in any part of this cortex will lead to *focal* weakness in that representative area in the contralateral body. As the axons from the motor cortex course down through the internal capsule and brainstem, they bundle close together. Unfortunately, a bundle of axons that is subjected to even a small lesion can lead to dramatic weakness in all represented areas, also in the contralateral body. The axons decussate in the medulla to fall into the corticospinal tracts in the lateral spinal cord until they reach the appropriate spinal level to create a synapse on the spinal motor neuron (Fig. 4-2).

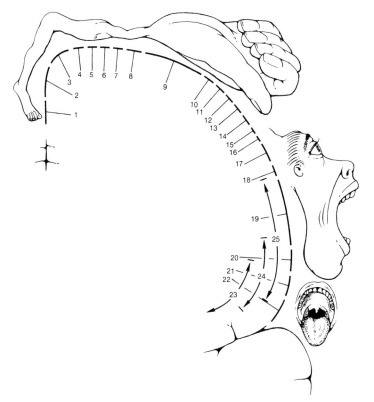

FIGURE 4-1: **Homunculus.** The homunculus is a representative map of the motor cortex that graphically shows the layout of the innervating motor areas from the legs in the sagittal sinus to the face on the inferolateral frontal lobe.

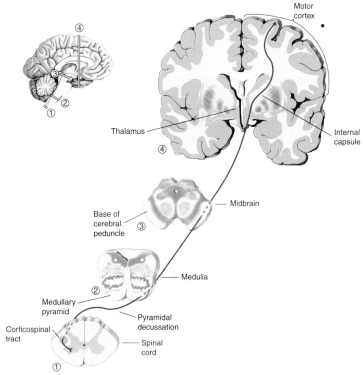

FIGURE 4-2: **The Corticospinal Tract.** The course of the corticospinal tract starts in the motor cortex where alpha motor neurons project their long axons down through the subcortical white matter, around the thalamus and into the brainstem where they decussate before tracking down the spinal cord. The first synapse occurs at the exit level of the spinal cord on either the lower motor neuron itself or interneurons in proximity. Adapted from Bear MF, Connors BW, and Parasido, MA. *Neuroscience - Exploring the Brain,* 2nd Ed. Philadelphia: Lippincott Williams & Wilkins, 2001.

A lesion in the corticospinal tract will cause weakness in the ipsilateral body at the level of lesion and below. For example, a lesion at T7 will cause weakness of the abdominal muscles, back, and legs. A specific lesion of the spinal motor neurons, as occurs in amyotrophic lateral sclerosis (ALS), a motor neuron disease, causes weakness of the limbs subserved by those neurons. The spinal motor neurons project their axons out of the central nervous system into the peripheral nervous system until they reach their target neuromuscular junction.

Dysfunction of the peripheral motor nerves, from Guillain-Barré syndrome, for example, will lead to weakness of the muscle to which the nerve is connected. Peripheral motor nerves can be focally affected (e.g., by injury) or systemically affected (e.g., in Guillain-Barré syndrome).

At the neuromuscular junction, acetylcholine is released by the presynaptic terminal in response to calcium influx, which can be blocked by circulating pathologic antibodies. The acetylcholine normally diffuses across the neuromuscular junction to bind to acetylcholine receptors on the muscles. However, if pathologic circulating antibodies block the acetylcholine receptors, the patient will feel weak. Weakness at the neuromuscular junction due to circulating pathologic antibodies causes generalized weakness rather than focal weakness because the circulating antibodies have access to all of the neuromuscular junctions in the body.

Finally, dysfunction of the muscle itself causes weakness. Muscles are susceptible to trauma, inflammation, infection, and deconditioning, among other pathologies.

Epidemiology

Weakness is a broad complaint that encompasses many different types of disease whose epidemiology varies widely.

ACUTE MANAGEMENT AND WORKUP

The acute management and workup of weakness always starts with ruling out life-threatening conditions. The life-threatening causes of acute weakness include hemorrhagic and ischemic stroke, subdural hematoma, focal seizures, spinal cord compression, and rhabdomyolysis. These conditions must be diagnosed early to prevent ongoing damage.

The First 15 Minutes

The first 15 minutes of your evaluation of a patient presenting with weakness should be focused on ruling out life-threatening conditions and stabilizing the patient. Even if your patient appears comfortably stable when you first arrive, you would be wise to think about the possible life-threatening conditions that could quickly present themselves. For example, an intracranial hemorrhage may initially present with sudden weakness in one limb, but with continued bleeding, may rapidly evolve into seizure, coma, or death.

Initial Assessment

As with every patient, the ABCs must be secured first as they are critical to life: airway, breathing, and circulation. The emergency room staff are adept at managing the ABCs of your patient, but it should still be the first thing you do as well. Assuming your patient is resting comfortably, breathing without distress, and not bleeding out, you can begin the initial workup for weakness.

For focal weakness, the initial assessment should focus on ruling out a life-threatening intracranial pathology, such as hemorrhagic or ischemic stroke. A noncontrast CT of the head is the best way to look for blood in the brain or dura. CT scans can detect an acute *ischemic* stroke only if the event occurred at least 6 hours previously. Otherwise, if you highly suspect an acute ischemic stroke that occurred within the 6 past hours, an emergent MRI should be obtained with the help of your senior resident.

At the same time that intracranial pathology is ruled out, spinal cord pathologies should be ruled out as well. Any history of trauma, falls, "found down by family or emergency medical service (EMS)," car accidents, or sports injuries should prompt the placement of a cervical collar and imaging of the spine. Your colleagues in neurosurgery should be notified immediately about any patient whose cause of weakness is acute spinal cord pathology, intracranial hemorrhage, subdural hematoma, or epidural hematoma. Finally, consider ordering a creatine kinase to rule out acute rhabdomyolysis if you discover exquisite tenderness on palpation of muscles, and a history of generalized weakness and darkened urine.

When you are reassured that your patient is not suffering from a life-threatening condition that led to the chief complaint of weakness, you can take a deep breath and begin a careful workup.

Admission Criteria and Level of Care Criteria

Obviously, if the initial workup reveals any of the life-threatening conditions you were concerned about in the initial workup, the patient should be considered for admission to the intensive care unit. At this point, you should involve your senior resident, fellow, or attending.

On the other end of the spectrum is the patient who presents with acute weakness that has already completely resolved. For these patients, if you cannot reliably rule out transient ischemic attack (TIA) by history (the patient's physical should be normal by definition), the patient will need to be admitted for TIA evaluation. Multiple studies have shown that hospitalization for TIA workup and treatment of stroke risk factors leads to a reduced risk of subsequent stroke.

If your patient's weakness is not owing to a life-threatening condition and is not completely resolved, admission to the neurology service should be considered under the following conditions:

- The patient's weakness is worsening.
- The cause of the weakness is unknown and may worsen.
- The weakness is caused by a known condition that may worsen at home in the near future.
- The treatment requires intensive therapy, such as intravenous medications.
- The patient is unsafe to return home because of the new weakness.

The First 24 Hours

In the first 24 hours of admission, the goal is to obtain all testing needed to help make the diagnosis and, if possible, to begin treatment.

History

There are three main aspects of the history that are important in assessing weakness: (i) the area of the body involved, (ii) the speed of the onset and the time of duration, and (iii) other symptoms the patient may be experiencing.

In determining the area of the body involved, ask the patient exactly what part (or parts) of the body is weak and ask for specific examples about how he noticed the weakness impacting his life. For example, if a patient complains about right leg weakness, ask about involvement of the foot, ankle, and knee; also ask if the weakness has limited the patient's walking, has resulted in difficulty climbing stairs, and has resulted in the patient's experiencing near-falls. Ask about all areas involved. Sometimes a patient may tell you about his very weak right arm but neglect to mention that the right leg is weak too because it is not as weak as the arm. Look for patterns that will help you localize the lesion. For example, if a patient complains of right arm and leg weakness, make sure you ask about facial involvement. Right facial weakness, left facial weakness, or no facial weakness each has significant impact on the localization of this pattern of weakness.

The second major aspect of the history that is important in assessing weakness is the time course. Was the onset of the weakness sudden? Did it stutter at first and then stay weak? Was the patient weak yesterday, then return to normal, and is weak again today? Did the weakness progress over hours, days, or weeks? Does it relapse and remit? If the weakness improved by the time you see the patient, ask about the time course of improvement. Was the improvement sudden or gradual? The answers to these questions will be important in narrowing your differential diagnosis.

Finally, the third major aspect of the history that is important to ask about is the association of other symptoms. Other symptoms may provide important clues to both the localization and the etiology. In particular, ask about functions that co-localize with weakness at each level of the neuroaxis:

- *Cortex.* Does the patient complain of language, memory, or cognitive difficulties?
- *Subcortex.* Is there numbness in the same distribution as the weakness?
- *Thalamus.* Trick question! Pure thalamic dysfunction should not cause weakness because motor relays pass *around* the thalamus.
- *Brainstem.* Does the patient complain of diplopia, dysphagia, dysarthria, vertigo, or hearing difficulties?
- *Spinal cord.* Is there numbness in the distribution *contralateral* to the weakness? Is there bowel and bladder involvement?

- *Peripheral nerves.* Does the weakness involve the entire body? Was there a history of injury to one particular limb that may have involved the nerve?

> ### CLINICAL PEARL
>
> *A typical pattern of weakness caused by a peripheral nerve lesion that is commonly confused for a stroke is isolated radial nerve palsy, which causes weakness of the extensor muscles of the hands and fingers.*

- *Neuromuscular junction.* Is there a history of previously diagnosed myasthenia gravis or lung cancer that may suggest the presence of circulating antibodies?
- *Muscle.* Is there a history of vigorous exercise, trauma, or tenderness of muscles? Is there a history of dark-colored urine?

Do not forget to document relevant aspects of the past medical history, social history, and family history. For example, does the patient have a past medical history of vasculitis or cancer that may increase stroke risk? Smoking increases stroke risk, and statin drugs may cause muscular pains and weakness. A family history of muscular dystrophy would be an obvious relevant aspect of the history to mention on rounds.

Physical Examination

As with every patient, a complete physical exam should precede the neurologic exam. Pay special attention to the head and neck for evidence of trauma, listen for carotid bruits, and palpate the limb muscles to assess for tenderness.

A complete neurologic exam follows the general physical exam. The following are the critical areas to focus on:

- *Mental status.* Test for impairments in cognitive, memory, and language function that may localize a focal lesion to the cerebral cortex. Also, note that systemic metabolic disturbances in patients with poor neurologic reserve may also cause generalized weakness.
- *Cranial nerves.* Test all cranial nerves to reassure your senior resident that a brainstem pathology will not eminently lead to death or to a locked-in state. This cannot be overemphasized. Check for pupillary function, dysconjugate eye deviation, ptosis, facial symmetry and strength, hearing and balance, palate elevation, and tongue strength. If there are any deficits in cranial nerves associated with focal weakness, consider this a brainstem pathologic emergency and immediately involve your senior resident or attending. Do not wait to alert the team about brainstem dysfunction

because whatever may have caused this particular lesion may presently cause permanent devastating damage or death.

- *Motor function*. First make a note of differences in tone and bulk between the affected and unaffected muscles; acute weakness will not cause changes in bulk, but the muscle tone may be increased or decreased. As best as you can, in testing, isolate each muscle in the affected limb or body part. Begin with the limb in the maximally extended position to test extensor strength or in a maximally flexed position to test flexor strength, and apply consistent counterforce for at least a few seconds. If there is no apparent weakness on examination despite the patient's complaint, the weakness may be too subtle to test by confrontation. In that case, you may test for pronator drift and orbit. Ask the patient to hold his or her arms out, and, with palms up and fingers spread apart, ask the patient to close his or her eyes. Look for *pronation*, a turning inward of the palms. Pronation is evidence for upper motor neuron weakness (from the brain to the spinothalamic tract). To test orbit, ask the patient to spin his or her arms around each other like a boxer. The stronger arm will eventually move faster around the weaker arm.

- *Sensation*. Test for changes in soft touch, pinprick, vibration, and temperature in the weak areas and compare them to the normal areas. A combined sensory/motor deficit carries a very different differential diagnosis.

- *Reflexes*. Reflexes are the most objective exam results. Test for reflexes, paying special attention to the difference in the weak limbs compared to the normal limbs. Increased reflexes are suggested of chronic upper motor neuron denervation whereas decreased reflexes may reflect a very acute lower motor neuron weakness.

- *Coordination*. Sometimes people say they are weak but really mean dizzy, light-headed, or incoordinated. Test for these functions to exclude a miscommunication.

- *Gait*. Weakness in the legs should result in impaired gait, so make sure your patient does not fall while you are testing him or her. In patients with complaints of focal weakness in the legs, pay attention to how the patient's ankles and knees move.

Labs and Tests to Consider

There are many blood tests that may be useful in your weakness workup, but only a few are necessary. Table 4-1 lists common labs to order categorized by localization.

Key Diagnostic Labs and Tests

Because there are many causes of weakness, lab testing should not include all of those listed in Table 4-1. Rather, your workup should be focused by localization. If you suspect a problem in the brain, for example, there is little value in sending for anti-acetylcholine antibodies found in neuromuscular

TABLE 4-1

Key Diagnostic Labs and Tests for Weakness Workup

Localization	Key Labs
Brain	Stroke-risk stratification labs: TSH, RPR, ESR, homocysteine, lipid profile.
Spinal cord	Lumbar puncture to rule out infection and inflammation; remember to send for cell counts in two separate tubes to account for possible blood contamination from a traumatic tap.
Peripheral nerves	Hemoglobin A1c, ESR, CRP
Neuromuscular junction	Anti–acetylcholine receptor antibodies; anti-MUSK (muscle-specific kinase) antibodies, anti–voltage-gated calcium channel antibodies.
Muscle	Creatine kinase, aldolase

TSH, thyroid-stimulating hormone; RPR, rapid plasmin reagent; ESR, erythrocyte sedimentation rate; CRP, C-reactive protein.

disease. Conversely, if you suspect a primary muscle disease, a spinal tap may be unnecessary.

Imaging and Ancillary Testing

Ancillary tests will prove very useful in your workup. Before ordering any of these expensive studies, you should already expect the abnormality. The imaging test is designed to *confirm* your localization, not *create* it. See Table 4-2 for key imaging tests that can be used to help determine the causes of patient weakness.

Assessment

As always, the assessment includes three key parts:

1. *A succinct, summary sentence that includes the most important aspects of the history, physical, and tests.* A succinct summary should include the key features of the history, physical, and ancillary testing, and should not be more than two or three sentences. It should be composed in a way that supports your proposed localization and differential diagnosis (information to be provided in later sections).

TABLE 4-2

Key Imaging Tests and Rationales for Testing

Test	Rationale
Noncontrast head computed tomography (CT)	Rule out (r/o) intracranial hemorrhage from stroke or subarachnoid hemorrhage, subdural hemorrhage from trauma, previous strokes, and hydrocephalus.
Magnetic resonance imaging (MRI) of head	R/o acute ischemic stroke, tumors, inflammation such as multiple sclerosis, infection such as empyema, and trauma.
Electroencephalogram (EEG)	R/o ongoing or intermittent seizure activity.
Electromyogram (EMG) and nerve conduction study (NCS)	NCS will rule out neuropathic pathologies such as peripheral demyelination or axonal damage; EMG will rule out muscle pathology such as inflammation (myositis) or neuromuscular junction dysfunction. EMG/NCS can yield false-negative results early in the disease process and should be repeated if weakness lasts >2 weeks for an optimal study.

2. *Localization.* Localization is a feature unique and important to neurology. Logical thinking of the patient's history and physical should narrow down the location of the lesion; ancillary testing will help confirm your localization. The key features of weakness that localize to a particular level of the nervous system are the following:

   • Cortex. Weakness should be associated with other cortical functions, such as language, memory, and cognition. However, there are many cases of isolated weakness caused by cortical lesions. When localizing cortical lesions, consider the homunculus in Figure 4–1. Weakness of the leg and face, without involvement of the arm, *could not* logically localize to one lesion in the cortex. In general, it is good practice to rule out a cortical lesion if there is any suspicion. An electroencephalogram (EEG) and MRI of the brain, with contrast, should be obtained to specifically rule out a cortical cause.

   • *Subcortex.* Weakness should present in the particular pattern represented by the organization of white matter fibers coursing from the cortex to the brainstem through the internal capsule. The organization of motor axons is arranged in the following order:

- Contralateral and ipsilateral facial axons most medially
- Contralateral arms and thorax next to the face
- Contralateral legs most laterally

These motor fibers are closely opposed to sensory fibers subserving the contralateral body. Thus, a typical subcortical lesion results in weakness of the contralateral face (but sparing the upper face because of bilateral innervation) and the arm and leg, which is often associated with sensory loss in the same distribution. Subcortical structures are packed tightly and thus are susceptible to even small lesions.

CLINICAL PEARL

A stroke affecting the face, arm, and leg on one side almost always involves the subcortical white matter.

Figure 4-3 outlines a simple algorithm for sorting out a cortical versus subcortical lesion based on physical exam.

- *Brainstem.* Weakness may be associated with cranial nerve palsies and crossed findings. Cranial nerve palsies can cause diplopia and dysconjugate gaze, facial weakness (upper *and* lower face) ipsilateral to the lesion, vertigo, dysarthria, and tongue deviation. Crossed findings of weakness in the ipsilateral face plus contralateral body localizes to the brainstem where facial motor axons have crossed but the body motor axons have not. Remember, cranial nerve palsies and crossed findings suggesting brainstem pathology is an emergency! Whatever caused the patient's current brainstem findings may quickly worsen to cause permanent disability or death.
- *Spinal cord.* The key to localizing spinal cord pathology lies in the discovery of a sensory level. If you discover on sensory examination that sensation is altered below a certain spinal level (either unilateral or bilateral sensory loss), spinal cord pathology moves to the top of your list. Also unique to the spinal cord is the apposed arrangement of ipsilateral sensory fibers going to the brain from the body with contralateral motor fibers that are coming down from the brain to the body. Thus, if you discover sensory loss in the distribution opposite the weakness, such as sensory loss of the right arm with weakness of the left arm, that pattern localizes to the spinal cord.
- *Peripheral nerves.* The two big clues that suggest weakness because of peripheral nerves are diffuse, generalized weakness and/or traumatic

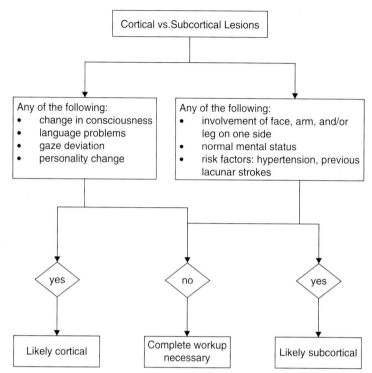

FIGURE 4-3: A basic algorithm for differentiating a cortical versus subcortical lesion based solely on history and physical exam.

injury to a single peripheral nerve. Weakness owing to peripheral nerve involvement is common because of systemic abnormalities such as medication toxicity that affects all peripheral nerves, equally leading to generalized weakness. Early in the course, the longest nerves may be affected distally first. That is because the longest nerves are the most susceptible to injury given the distance from the reparative machinery in the cell body.

• *Neuromuscular junction.* Similar to peripheral nerve lesions, weakness owing to involvement of the neuromuscular junction is generalized. The eyelids are particularly sensitive to anti-MUSK antibodies, and proximal muscles may be more affected by anti–acetylcholine receptor antibodies, especially with repetitive movements. In contrast, antibodies against the presynaptic voltage-gated potassium channel seen in Eaton-Lambert syndrome leads to increased strength with repeated use. In other words, patients with myasthenia gravis get more fatigued with repetitive muscle use, whereas patients with Eaton-Lambert get stronger with repetitive muscle use.

• *Muscle.* In the absence of trauma, muscle disease is usually systemic and causes generalized weakness. Muscle tenderness, elevated creatine kinase and aldolase levels, and electromyogram (EMG) abnormalities are big clues to muscle localization.

   After considering the localization, you may find that you need additional testing to narrow down the location of the lesion.

3. *Differential diagnosis.* The differential diagnosis and treatment are particular to the localization. Table 4-3 lists the common differential diagnosis items for each level of the nervous system, as well as the features of each etiology.

Treatment

The field of neurology is reaching the point that effective treatment for many previously untreatable neurologic illnesses is now available. One of the emerging new therapies in neurology is the thrombolysing drug tissue plasminogen activation (tPA) for use in acute ischemic stroke. If the time of onset of symptoms can be confirmed to have started within 3 hours of presentation to the emergency room, thrombolysis with intravenous tPA can be considered. In cases of uncertain time of onset, the time *last seen normal* is considered the time of onset because if a patient wakes up with a stroke, the ischemic event could have happened early in the night. Administration of intravenous tPA to patients with strokes older than 3 hours imposes an excessive risk of intracranial hemorrhage and is therefore contraindicated. An exception to this 3-hour rule is permitted at hospitals where intra-arterial tPA by catheterization of the thrombosed cerebral artery can be performed within 6 hours of symptom onset or the time last seen normal. Two studies have shown a modest benefit in long-term outcome using tPA instead of aspirin, but the decision to use tPA in an acute ischemic stroke should always be confirmed by the attending physician because of the risk of hemorrhage in the area of the stroke caused by thrombolysis.

Table 4-4 lists all of the treatments for the causes listed in Table 4-3.

EXTENDED INHOSPITAL MANAGEMENT

Workup typically takes up to 24 to 48 hours, depending on the tests that are ordered. Empiric therapy may be initiated, especially if infection is suspected.

Physical therapy is almost universally helpful. A physical therapist should be consulted to evaluate and suggest a physical therapy plan to improve strength in the affected areas.

TABLE 4-3
Differential Diagnosis by Localization

Level of the Nervous System	Etiology	Features
Cortex	Ischemic stroke	Very common, especially in patients with stroke risk factors: smoking, age, hypertension, diabetes, hypercholesterolemia. MRI is positive for stroke within 20 minutes of event; >99% sensitive. *Embolic* strokes are more common in cortex.
	Hemorrhagic stroke	Easily visible on noncontrast head CT; common in patients with hypertension, cerebral amyloid angiopathy; may cause seizures.
	Tumor	Slow onset, associated with seizures; edema seen on CT, MRI with contrast confirms the diagnosis.
	Seizure	Postictal weakness is called Todd's paralysis; should resolve within 24 hours.
	Migraine	Familial hemiplegic migraine causes weakness of body contralateral to headache.
	Infection/ empyema	Associated with fevers, leukocytosis, elevated CSF white cell count, positive Gram stain; visible on MRI and edema seen on CT.
	Inflammation	Rheumatologic diseases such as lupus can involve the cortex. MS variants occasionally involve the cortex.

(continued)

TABLE 4-3

Differential Diagnosis by Localization (Continued)

Level of the Nervous System	Etiology	Features
Subcortex	Ischemic stroke	*Thrombotic* ischemic strokes are *very* common in the subcortex; some are asymptomatic. Same stroke risk factors as cortical strokes.
	Hemorrhagic strokes	The subcortex is the most common location of hypertensive hemorrhagic strokes.
	Multiple sclerosis (MS)	White matter inflammatory disease associated with oligoclonal bands in CSF and MRI enhancement; rarely seen in patients >50 years old.
Brainstem	Ischemic stroke	Posterior circulation involvement of the vertebral and basilar arteries are seen in all age groups.
	Hemorrhagic strokes	Devastating, life-threatening emergency. Easily visible on CT.
	Bell's palsy	Must be associated with loss of taste on ipsilateral tongue and increased ipsilateral echogenicity of sounds.
	Lyme disease	History of tick bite and target rash; associated with fevers, arthritis; commonly affects multiple cranial nerves. Diagnosed by CSF lyme antibody titer.

TABLE 4-3

Differential Diagnosis by Localization (Continued)

Level of the Nervous System	Etiology	Features
	Sarcoidosis	Predilection for the brainstem; involves multiple bilateral cranial nerves; enhanced by MRI.
	Tuberculosis	Predilection for the brainstem in populations from third world countries.
Spinal cord	Cord compression	Associated with history of degenerative disc disease and trauma; MRI shows cord signal hyperintensity.
	Transverse myelitis/ MS	Small areas of demyelination of white matter seen in MS, longer lesions associated with neuromyelitis optica.
	Epidural abscess	Common in intravenous drug abusers; associated with fevers, exquisite back tenderness.
	Motor neuron disease (ALS)	Presents with muscle fasciculation and atrophy; EMG shows denervation and recruitment.
Peripheral nerves	Guillain-Barré syndrome	Ascending paralysis, rare sensory involvement; NCS shows peripheral demyelination.
	Chronic inflammatory demyelinating polyneuropathy	Recurrent episodes of peripheral demyelination.
	Rheumatologic diseases	Focal inflammation of nerves e.g. Churg-Strauss syndrome.

(continued)

TABLE 4-3

Differential Diagnosis by Localization (Continued)

Level of the Nervous System	Etiology	Features
Neuromuscular junction	Myasthenia gravis	Fatigable generalized weakness, eye and eyelid involvement are common; diagnosed by repetitive stimulation EMG, presence of circulating antibodies.
	Eaton-Lambert syndrome	Associated with small cell lung cancer; paraneoplastic process.
	Botulinum toxicity	History of exposure to contaminated foods such as unprocessed honey.
Muscle	Polymyositis	Inflammation of muscles of unknown cause; markedly elevated CK levels; affects large prominal muscles preferentially.
	Steroid myopathy	History of prolonged steroid use (>3 months) associated with proximal muscle weakness.
	Inclusion body myositis	Chronic inflammatory disease in older populations with preferential distal muscle involvement; muscle biopsy is gold standard for diagnosis.
	Deconditioning	History of prolonged muscle disuse and atrophy. Common in institutionalized patients.
	Genetic	Young patients with a family history of muscular dystrophy or glycogen storage diseases; too numerous to list . . .

CSF, cerebrospinal fluid; EMG, electromyogram.

TABLE 4-4

Treatment for Neurologic Diseases That
Cause Weakness

Level of the Nervous System	Etiology	Treatment
Cortex	Ischemic stroke	If within 3–6 hours of onset of stroke, thrombolysis and/or daily aspirin plus rehabilitation. For stroke recurrence, reduce stroke risk factors: hypertension, diabetes, hypercholesterolemia, smoking.
	Hemorrhagic stroke	Control blood pressure <180 mm Hg systolic; correct coagulopathy if present.
	Tumor	Neurosurgical consultation, oncologic consultation.
	Seizure	Many available treatments based on seizure type. See Treatment section in Chapter 6, Convulsions.
	Migraine	Many available treatments. See Treatment section in Chapter 10, Headache.
	Infection/empyema	Antibiotics, possible surgical drainage.
	Inflammation	Steroids in the acute period; stronger immunosuppressants may be necessary.
Subcortex	Ischemic stroke	See Cortex.
	Hemorrhagic strokes	See Cortex.

(continued)

TABLE 4-4

Treatment for Neurologic Diseases That Cause Weakness (Continued)

Level of the Nervous System	Etiology	Treatment
	Multiple sclerosis	Steroids in the acute period; long-term treatment with beta-interferons or glatiramer acetate.
Brainstem	Ischemic stroke	See Cortex.
	Hemorrhagic strokes	See Cortex.
	Bell's palsy	Prednisone taper for 2 weeks; consider adding 1 week of valacyclovir therapy (evidence pending).
	Lyme disease	Intravenous ceftriaxone for 3 weeks.
	Sarcoidosis	Low-dose steroids; long-term therapy with steroid-sparing immunosuppressants.
	Tuberculosis (TB)	Four-drug TB therapy: isoniazid, rifampin, pyrazinamide, and ethambutol for 6–18 months.
Spinal cord	Cord compression	In the hyperacute period (within 4 hours of injury), high-dose steroids: 30 mg/kg methylprednisone intravenously; emergent surgical intervention.
	Transverse myelitis/ multiple sclerosis (MS)	Steroids in the acute period; stronger immunosuppressants may be necessary.

TABLE 4-4

Treatment for Neurologic Diseases That Cause Weakness (Continued)

Level of the Nervous System	Etiology	Treatment
	Epidural abscess	Antibiotics, possible surgical drainage.
	Motor neuron disease (ALS)	Riluzole may extend life for a few months.
Peripheral nerves	Guillain-Barré syndrome	Intravenous gamma globulin.
	Chronic inflammatory demyelinating polyneuropathy	Intravenous gamma globulin.
	Rheumatologic diseases	Immunosuppression
Neuromuscular junction	Myasthenia gravis	Combination of immunosuppression with steroid-sparing agents plus pyridostigmine for symptoms.
	Eaton-Lambert syndrome	Plasma exchange.
	Botulinum toxicity	Antitoxin is effective only within first 24 hours; antibiotics if gut is actively infected; supportive care until botulinum toxin is cleared.
Muscle	Polymyositis	Steroids in the acute period; stronger immunosuppressants may be necessary; physical therapy to improve recovery.

(continued)

TABLE 4-4

Treatment for Neurologic Diseases That Cause Weakness (Continued)

Level of the Nervous System	Etiology	Treatment
	Steroid myopathy	Cessation of steroids; physical therapy.
	Inclusion body myositis	No effective treatment is currently available.
	Deconditioning	Physical therapy.
	Genetic	Depends on the exact condition.

DISPOSITION

Discharge Goals

The goals of discharge are threefold:

- Workup of the underlying etiology that caused weakness as well as identification of diagnosis
- Treatment of the underlying disorder
- Prevention of recurrence:
  - Successful prevention depends on the cause. For example, to prevent recurrence of ischemic stroke, the risk factors should be modified. Hemorrhagic strokes can be prevented by controlling hypertension. The risk of an exacerbation of multiple sclerosis can be reduced with beta-interferons or glatiramer acetate.

Outpatient Care

Outpatient follow-up is the single best intervention to prevent recurrence and should be arranged before the patient leaves the hospital. If available in your hospital or in your area, refer your patients for follow-up with a neurologic specialist. Neurologic specialties include the following:

- Stroke
- Neuro-oncology
- Epilepsy
- Headaches
- Neuroimmunology/neuroinfectious diseases (handles multiple sclerosis, infectious diseases, and diseases such as neurosarcoidosis)

- Neuromuscular (handles peripheral nerve, neuromuscular junction, and muscle diseases)

WHAT YOU NEED TO REMEMBER

- Weakness can be focal or generalized. Focal weakness can localize to any level of the neuroaxis, but generalized weakness is generally caused by peripheral nerve, neuromuscular junction, or muscle disease.
- Evaluation and workup of acute weakness should start with ruling out life-threatening conditions. Anything that localizes to the brain, especially the brainstem, should be considered an emergency.
- The three main aspects of the history in patients with weakness are identification of the exact body parts affected, the time course of onset and duration, and other symptoms associated with the weakness.
- The physical exam should not only focus on the area of weakness but must be complete to be able to localize the lesion correctly. Ancillary tests, such as MRI, serve to confirm your localization.
- The differential diagnosis of weakness is specific to the localization within the neuroaxis, and the treatment is specific to the cause.

SUGGESTED READINGS

Bradley WG, Daroff RB, Fenichel G, et al. *Neurology in Clinical Practice.* Amsterdam, the Netherlands: Elsevier, 2004.

Greenberg D, Aminoff MJ, Simon RP. *Clinical Neurology.* 5th Ed. New York: McGraw-Hill/Appleton & Lange, 2002.

Tingling and Numbness

OVERVIEW

Definition and Pathophysiology

Tingling is a symptom the patient feels when sensation is reduced or different. Common descriptions of tingling include "pins and needles," "like my arm went to sleep," and "like my skin is thick." Numbness is a sign that sensation is abnormal; it is usually discovered on neurologic examination. Tingling and numbness can be present together or alone in many different situations, from the most harmless conditions to the most severe.

Sensation is carried by dorsal root ganglia sensory axons from the skin and viscera to the dorsal spinal cord where they synapse and cross either to the spinothalamic tract (touch, temperature) or the dorsal columns (vibration, proprioception). These tracts course up through the brainstem and synapse in the thalamus on their way up to the sensory cortex. A lesion at any point along the sensory tract from the peripheral nerves to the sensory cortex may present with tingling and/or numbness. Many different types of lesions can affect sensory nerves from traumatic nerve damage, medication toxicity, chemotherapies, diabetes, spinal cord injury, and tumors, to name a few.

Epidemiology

Numbness and tingling can be signs of other, more serious common neurologic diseases such as stroke and multiple sclerosis. These diseases additionally present with other signs and symptoms, but, on rare occasion, a sensory abnormality is the only finding. Numbness and tingling may also represent primary sensory nerve dysfunction when other neurologic signs and symptoms, such as weakness, are absent. These conditions are very common and include mild to moderate diabetic neuropathy, HIV sensory neuropathy, and vitamin B12 deficiency. Finally, but uncommon, there are patients whose primary complaint is numbness and tingling in which no primary nerve dysfunction and no other neurologic diseases are found.

ACUTE MANAGEMENT AND WORKUP

Most people can recall waking up with a numb arm or shaking off a foot that has "fallen asleep." These episodes usually do not worry people; if an individual does happen to present to the triage nurse in the emergency room with one of these complaints, the complaint usually resolves by the time you see the patient. However, numbness and tingling that is different from one of the mentioned typical episodes should be taken seriously, especially if the patient has risk factors for developing other diseases. For example, a patient with stroke risk factors of hypertension and diabetes should be worked up for stroke if she develops an acute onset of left-sided numbness and tingling. In general, it is better to always take seriously any new onset of numbness and tingling until a cause is discovered.

The First 15 Minutes

The first 15 minutes of your evaluation of a patient with a primary complaint of numbness and tingling is to rule out a life-threatening neurologic condition. These include stroke, intracranial hemorrhage, meningitis or encephalitis, seizure, and trauma.

Initial Assessment

Follow these quick steps in first evaluating any patient with new tingling and/or numbness:

1. *Check the patient's vital signs.* Make sure the oxygen saturation is at baseline or higher. Make sure the patient is breathing comfortably. Hyperventilation can cause tingling in the fingertips and around the lips.
2. *Look for associated neurologic signs and symptoms.* Does the patient have sensory complaints in isolation or are there other problems as well? If the patient has mental status changes, cranial nerve deficits, or weakness, the problem may be life threatening. If your resident knows only about the sensory complaints, be sure to let him or her know about your other findings right away.
3. *Look for obvious emergent signs that require rapid attention*:
   • Decreased responsiveness
   • Asymmetric, dilated, unreactive pupils or symmetric pinpoint pupils
   • Hemiparesis or neglect, as seen when the patient totally ignores everything on her left side, including you, until you move to her right side.
   • Respiratory distress
   • Blood sugar <60 mg/dL
   • Seizure activity

If you find any of the conditions just listed, the sensory complaint is now a minor component of a much bigger problem and you must call your resident or attending.

Admission Criteria and Level of Care Criteria

The need to admit a patient with a sensory chief complaint depends largely on the suspected cause of the complaint. For example, if there is sensory loss caused by new stroke, the patient will be admitted to work up the stroke. On the other hand, if there is ongoing sensory loss in a patient with poorly controlled diabetes, the patient may be more effectively treated as an outpatient. If the cause cannot be determined on the initial evaluation, it will be important to consider the acuity of the symptoms. If the patient has recent-onset and progressive symptoms, consider that his or her condition will continue to worsen and that the patient requires admission for further evaluation and monitoring.

The First 24 Hours

Workup for tingling and/or numbness can be frustrating because the location and severity of symptoms often fluctuate. In patients with a chief complaint of tingling and/or numbness, it is common that findings on the student's exam are different from the exam elicited by the attending on rounds the next morning. Focus on the patient's history and the aspects of the physical exam that are easily reproducible.

History

The interpretation of sensory input is accomplished by a complex set of nervous system components. Because of this, your historical understanding of the patient's sensory complaints can provide much information about the possible causes of those complaints. Keep in mind that sensory dysfunction can be a result of a lesion(s) at multiple levels of the nervous system: sensory cortex, thalamus, brainstem, spinal cord, nerve root, nerve plexus, or peripheral nerve.

Your goals in evaluating a patient with a chief complaint of sensory deficits include the following:

1. *Obtain a precise description of the patient's symptoms.* Numbness is a vague term that means different things to different people. To a medical student or neurologist, *numb* might indicate a decreased perception or lack of sensation. To a patient, however, *numb* can often mean an altered sensation, such as a burning sensation. There are many ways in which sensation can be altered. Most commonly, the patient will describe tingling, and may interchangeably use the terms tingling and numbness. To a medical student or neurologist, tingling is usually termed *paresthesias*. Often, paresthesias and numbness will occur together, although the patient may be aware of only the paresthesias.

You will also want to know if the patient is experiencing associated pain. If so, how does the patient describe the pain? Sharp, shooting, and/or burning pain is often associated with injury to the peripheral nervous system. Other important terms to be aware of include *hyperesthesia* (increased sensitivity to any stimulation), *dysesthesia* (distortion of sensation, usually such that a normal stimulus produces an unpleasant response), and *allodynia* (pain owing to a stimulus that does not normally produce pain).

2. *Determine the neuroanatomic location of the sensory complaints.* When localizing sensory complaints, start with the cortical level and move down the nervous system.

> ### CLINICAL PEARL
>
> *Hemisensory complaints involving the face, arm, trunk, and leg are likely to represent an intracranial pathology. If sensory complaints are entirely located below a certain level—for example, midchest (with normal sensation above the level), the lesion probably involves the spinal cord. If the sensory complaints are confined to one or more specific large or small "patches" on the body, it could indicate a lesion of one or more nerve roots or peripheral nerves, depending on the exact location of the patch(es). If the sensory complaints are symmetric and distal, affecting the feet and subsequently the lower legs followed by the hands and the more proximal legs, the problem is likely diffusely affecting the distal nerves in a so-called stocking-glove pattern.*

3. *Determine if there are associated symptoms.* There are relatively few specific conditions that cause sensory complaints in isolation. Such conditions must involve only the sensory nerves or pathways while sparing all other components of the nervous system, such as the peripheral motor neurons. Sensory symptoms in isolation might also suggest a non-neurologic cause of the complaints, such as hyperventilation or hypoventilation caused by cardiorespiratory conditions or anxiety. Be careful, however, because associated sensory symptoms (or signs) may be subtle or unimportant to the patient, or may appear subsequent to initial sensory involvement. Performing a thorough neurologic exam may allow you to pick up subtle weakness or cranial nerve deficits that will change where you localize the lesion.

4. *Identify the acuity of onset and rate of progression.* As with most complaints in neurology, you want to know how fast the symptom started and whether it has stayed exactly the same since onset or has spread to affect

a larger area of the body or progressed in intensity. The pattern of progression provides a clue to the cause. Acute-onset hemisensory loss should prompt you to consider a stroke as the cause rather than a brain tumor, which more likely will produce progressively worsening symptoms over days to weeks.

5. *Medications.* Many drugs are neurotoxic to the peripheral nervous system, leading predominantly to sensory complaints. The most common neurotoxic drugs include chemotherapeutic agents and antimicrobials. Symptoms of neurotoxicity usually occur after chronic use of the offending medication and may improve with discontinuation. Numbness and tingling are common side effects of many medications, even if they are not particularly neurotoxic, and the exact cause of the sensory adverse effect may be unknown. Consider this cause in the setting of a new medication or change in dose.

6. *Past medical history.* Make special note of the following:
   • Metabolic conditions that can affect the peripheral nerves, such as diabetes and renal failure
   • Cancer, for which the patient may be on neurotoxic treatments
   • HIV, because both the virus and the treatments for the virus can cause neurotoxicity
   • Stroke risk factors
   • Immunosuppression or other risk factors for infection
   • Known neurologic disease that could cause new sensory complaints, such as multiple sclerosis

7. *Family history.* Some conditions that affect primarily or solely sensory pathways are hereditary, such as the hereditary sensory neuropathies. However, these are rare conditions; familial conditions are much more likely to involve both sensory and motor nerves, as with Charcot-Marie-Tooth disease.

8. *Social history.* The second or third most common cause of a length-dependent peripheral neuropathy in the United States (after glucose intolerance and possibly medication neurotoxicity) is alcoholic neurotoxicity. Usually this requires chronic and heavy alcohol use, but high-functioning individuals may not admit the full extent of their alcohol use, and it may sometimes occur with relatively little alcohol use. Also obtain a history of occupational exposures, especially heavy metals such as arsenic and mercury, which may first present with numbness and tingling.

Physical Examination

Because various sensory modalities are subserved by specific tracts and nuclei with well-defined anatomic localization, a comprehensive examination can provide a wealth of information about the nature, location, and cause of a nervous system lesion. However, because the sensory systems are so complex, a truly comprehensive sensory exam could take, literally, hours

to perform. Keep in mind that sensation is entirely subjective and dependent on the patient's cooperation. Subjective sensory deficits are very common especially with pseudoneurologic symptoms. It is therefore important
to assess how reliable the patient is in reporting sensory findings to you as
you do your exam. You must know your sensory anatomy to know whether
the sensory findings that your patient reports make anatomic sense. You
should have an idea of what kind of sensory findings you expect based on
your history and the rest of your neurologic examination. Also, keep in mind
that sensory symptoms often precede sensory signs, so an unrevealing sensory examination may simply reflect that an underlying condition is still relatively early in its clinical course.

In general, you are looking for asymmetries; distal-to-proximal gradients;
or sensory loss in the distribution of a specific nerve, nerve root, or central
pattern of the spinal cord or brain.

Perform a complete general and neurologic exam. Because the sensory
exam is so subjective, subtle sensory findings are usually insignificant. For
example, if the patient reports 100% sensation on one side of the body and
95% sensation on the other side, you can usually interpret that finding as
equivalent to symmetric sensation.

Make sure to perform the following key parts of the exam:

- *Extremities*: Changes in color, temperature, and hair pattern can sometimes accompany peripheral neuropathies. A patient with severe numbness may develop significant ulcers, usually on the feet, without realizing
  it, because he or she does not feel the pain that would usually be associated with such an ulcer.
- *Neurologic status*. Make sure to evaluate the following:
  - If the patient has significant acute mental status changes, you must be
    quite concerned about his or her immediate health risks. Do not spend
    time on an extensive sensory examination. Make sure your resident
    knows the situation and that your patient is getting the assessment he or
    she needs.
  - Cranial nerves. An abnormality of the cranial nerves, sensory or other-
    wise, suggests the lesion is located in the brainstem or perhaps in the
    basal meninges.
  - Motor. Does the patient have motor findings to accompany his or her
    sensory complaints? Are both the motor and sensory findings on one
    side of the body? Is the patient weak in one leg and numb in the other
    leg? Does the patient have evidence of both sensory loss and weakness
    in a particular radicular or peripheral nerve distribution? Are sensory
    and motor deficits diffuse? Is there evidence of upper or lower motor
    neuron involvement?
  - Coordination. If the patient is clumsy, is it because he or she has diffi-
    culty with joint position sensation or weakness?

- *Sensory exam.*
  - Light touch perception is a very nonlocalizing sensation. It can be used for routine screening, such as to see if the patient notes an asymmetry of which he or she may not have been previously aware. It is generally not valuable in more detailed assessment of sensory function.
  - Pain and temperature sensations travel together in the contralaterally spinothalamic tracts. In other words, the pathways that subserve these sensory modalities cross immediately on entering the spinal cord. For example, numbness to temperature sensation on the left trunk and leg may suggest a lesion in the right spinal cord. Pain is usually assessed by pinprick, and temperature by a cool tuning fork.
  - Vibration and proprioception (position sense) travel together in the ipsilateral dorsal columns of the spinal cord. The pathways that subserve these modalities enter and ascend in the spinal cord without crossing until they reach the medulla. Thus, proprioceptive loss in the right lower extremity may suggest a lesion in the right spinal cord, especially if it is accompanied by weakness in the right lower extremity and numbness to temperature sensation in the left lower extremity. (This example is a classic constellation of signs and symptoms called *Brown-Sequard syndrome.*) Proprioception is assessed by evaluating the ability of the patient to discriminate slight movements of a joint, such as slight up and down movements of the great toe. When you move the patient's toe up or down, make sure he or she is not looking, and grasp the joint laterally so as not to provide pressure cues to the patient. Vibration is usually assessed with a tuning fork placed on a distal joint. The patient indicates when the sensation can no longer be felt, and this is compared to whether the examiner can still feel the vibration. A 128-hertz tuning fork is used. Do not try to use a 512-hertz tuning fork, which is meant for the hearing examination.
  - Corticosensory modalities require significant cortical processing. These can be tested if there is a concern for a lesion in the sensory cortex. *Stereognosis* refers to the ability of the patient to identify objects by touch, such as a coin placed in the patient's hand. *Graphesthesia* is the ability to recognize numbers drawn in the palm of the hand. *Double simultaneous stimulation* refers to the ability to recognize two stimuli applied simultaneously to different parts of the body. *Extinction* is a form of sensory neglect, usually representing a contralateral parietal lobe lesion, which occurs when a patient recognizes a sensory stimulus to one side of the body when it is applied independently, but not when it is applied together with a stimulus to the other side of the body. *Two-point discrimination* refers to the ability to discriminate two sensory stimuli that are close together. For example, if two ends of a paper clip are applied to the pad of the index finger, a normal subject can tell that he or she has been touched by two points

rather than one, as long as the two points are two millimeters apart or greater.

- The Romberg test is often done along with the gait exam but is actually a functional exam of sensation. The patient stands with his or her feet together and is observed to see if he or she can maintain balance with the eyes closed. Three systems are used to maintain balance—vision, proprioception, and vestibular apparatus—but only two are required. Eye closure removes vision. Maintenance of balance implies functionally intact proprioception and vestibular input. Loss of balance implies disruption to either proprioception or vestibular input, and usually means proprioceptive loss because vestibular loss is associated with other signs and symptoms such as dizziness. If the patient has difficulty maintaining balance with feet together and eyes open, the Romberg test is unreliable. This usually occurs when there is a vestibular or cerebellar lesion. Many students make the mistake of testing pronator drift simultaneously with the Romberg test. These two tests are completely unrelated and should not be tested simultaneously.

Labs and Tests to Consider

It is not necessary to order each test on every patient with tingling and/or numbness. Some of these tests cost thousands of dollars and should be obtained only if they will significantly contribute to making a diagnosis or treatment decision.

Key Diagnostic Labs and Tests

Lab testing for patients with numbness and tingling should be focused by the history and physical exam. For example, if your workup thus far found a sensory loss only in a radicular distribution, there is no need to test for systemic causes of neuropathy, such as diabetes. In contrast, if your exam is consistent with peripheral neuropathy preferentially targeting the distal extremities, you should focus on testing for systemic conditions such as diabetes rather than looking for a focal lesion in the lumbar spinal cord.

Table 5-1 list the laboratory tests and rationales to be used in your workup.

Imaging and Ancillary Testing

The two most useful ancillary tests for patients with suspected peripheral nerve problems are a nerve conduction study for the dysfunction of large, myelinated nerves, and a skin biopsy for small-fiber nerve dysfunction. For lesions that localize to the central nervous system, MRI provides the highest-quality image of the brain and spinal cord.

Table 5-2 lists the imaging tests and rationales to be used in your workup.

TABLE 5-1
Key Laboratory Tests and Rationales for Testing

Test	Rationale
Oral glucose tolerance test, hemoglobin A1c	Rule out (r/o) diabetes or impaired glucose tolerance.
RPR, vitamin B12	R/o syphilis or B12 deficiency, which can cause dorsal column dysfunction.
Anti-Hu, Yo, Ri; serum/urine protein electrophoresis	R/o malignancies, which can cause peripheral neuropathies.
ESR, CRP	R/o inflammatory processes, which can affect peripheral nerves.
HIV	This infection and associated conditions can cause both peripheral and central sensory lesions.
Heavy metals screen	Chronic arsenic, lead, and mercury exposure can present with neuropathy.
Lumbar puncture Tube 1: cell count + differential (1.5 mL). Look for WBC to indicate infection/inflammation and RBC for blood in the CNS. Sometimes elevated RBC in the first tube suggests a traumatic spinal tap procedure. Compare to the counts in tube 4. Tube 2: glucose, protein (1.5 mL). High protein is seen in Guillain-Barrésyndrome. Tube 3: Gram's stain, culture, PCRs if necessary, VDRL to rule out neurosyphilis (6 mL). Tube 4: cell count + differential (1.5 mL).	Only required if there is a specific question that it will answer: • R/o meningoradiculitis or other infectious or inflammatory cause of sensory complaints • R/o cytoalbuminologic dissociation, which is seen with Guillain-Barré syndrome

RPR, rapid plasmin reagin; ESR, erythrocyte sedimentation rate; CRP, C-reactive protein; WBC, white blood count; RBC, red blood count; CNS, central nervous system; PCRs, polymerase chain reactions; VDRL, Venereal Disease Research Laboratories [test].

TABLE 5-2
Key Imaging Tests and Rationales for Testing

Test	Rationale
Nerve conduction study	Rule out (r/o) primary nerve dysfunction of large fiber nerves.
Skin biopsy	R/o small fiber nerve injury, which can be missed by EMG/NCV (skin biopsy assessment for small fiber neuropathy is conducted only at select academic medical centers).
Noncontrast Head Computed Tomography (CT)	Urgently r/o intracranial processes such as acute stroke or hemorrhage, brain tumor, or other mass lesion.
Magnetic Resonance Imaging (MRI) of head. When possible, an MRI is the ideal imaging modality because of the quality of the images and the increased sensitivity to evaluate for stroke, small tumors, and inflammatory neurologic diseases. However, the downsides of MRI are that it takes a long time to perform (up to 1 hour depending on the type of MRI), there are usually long lines in the hospital so it take hours before your patient is scanned, MRIs of the brain are expensive compared to CT scans ($1,500–$2,400), patients with pacemakers cannot get MRIs, and patients who are claustrophobic may not tolerate lying in the MRI scanner.	R/o intracranial pathology, which may be missed by head CT such as acute stroke (<6 hours old) or multiple sclerosis.
MRI of spine	R/o epidural abscess, spinal cord lesion, herniated disc, or other structural lesion as the cause of sensory complaints.

Assessment

The assessment comprises three key parts:

- *A succinct, summary sentence that includes the most important aspects of the history, physical exam, and tests.* For example: "40-year-old woman without significant past medical history presents with 5–6 days of ascending numbness and paresthesias and 1–2 days of ascending weakness."
- *Localization.* Use the patient's history and your examination skills to figure out in which of the following locations the lesion might be: sensory cortex, thalamus, brainstem, spinal cord, nerve root, nerve plexus, or peripheral nerve.
- *Differential diagnosis.* The differential diagnosis and treatment are largely dependent on your localization, the associated neurologic and systemic signs and symptoms, and the time course of the illness:
  - *Sensory cortex, thalamus, and brainstem.* Stroke, TIA, parenchymal hemorrhage, subdural hematoma, brain tumor, brain abscess, and multiple sclerosis
  - *Spinal cord.* Herniated disc, degenerative joint disease, epidural abscess, demyelinating plaque, spinal cord infarct, and spinal cord tumor
  - *Nerve root.* Meningoradiculitis (infectious, inflammatory, or malignant)
  - *Nerve plexus.* Idiopathic, malignant, traumatic, and diabetic
  - *Peripheral nerve.* Diabetes, alcoholism, chemotherapeutic neurotoxicity, Guillain-Barré syndrome, hereditary neuropathy, such as Charcot-Marie-Tooth disorder, vasculitis, infections, such as HIV, paraneoplastic neuropathy, entrapment, such as carpal tunnel syndrome, and vitamin deficiencies, such as B12 deficiency

Treatment

The treatment of tingling and numbness obviously depends on the etiology. Until the cause is determined, all patients should receive the following treatments:

1. All patients should be monitored to make sure their condition remains stable while the assessment for etiology is ongoing.
2. Treatment of the specific underlying cause should be instituted as soon as that cause is determined.
3. Symptomatic treatment should be instituted as appropriate. If numbness and/or paresthesias are bothersome enough, it may be reasonable to try a neuropathic pain medication. The options include serotonin-norepinephrine reuptake inhibitors (SNRIs), tricyclic antidepressants, and antiepileptic drugs. Pregabalin, gabapentin, valproate, and carbamazepine probably have the best literature support among the antiepileptic drugs. There is no way in advance to know for sure

which one of these medications may provide a patient with benefit. They must simply be tried in a sequential manner until an effective one is found that provides the maximum possible benefit. It is important with each medication trial to start at a low dose and increase slowly to avoid side effects, but not to discontinue the medication until an adequate dose has been achieved for a long enough time period—such as 4 to 6 weeks. Otherwise, it is not truly a medication failure. It may not be possible to find a medicine that will provide complete symptom relief without any side effects. Based on the patient's personal preferences, he or she may have to accept some side effects to maximize symptom relief or alternatively to accept some symptoms to minimize side effects. It is also important to recognize that these treatments are much more effective at treating neuropathic pain than they are at treating numbness or paresthesias. To the extent that the patient's complaint is the latter rather than the former, these medications may not work. These medications do not help with nerve regeneration; they are unnecessary unless the patient receives adequate symptomatic benefit.

EXTENDED INHOSPITAL MANAGEMENT

Extended inhospital management depends on the suspected or diagnosed underlying cause. Patients with serious or life-threatening causes require close monitoring with frequent neurologic assessments and review of vital signs and respiratory function. Patients with chronic sensory complaints may have most or all of their evaluation performed as an outpatient.

DISPOSITION

Discharge Goals

The goals of discharge are the following:

• Exclusion of a serious or life-threatening cause for the sensory complaints
• Stabilization and institution of specific therapy if a serious cause is diagnosed
• Initiation of symptomatic management

Outpatient Care

Outpatient follow-up should be arranged *before* the patient leaves the hospital. Make sure the patient has realistic diagnostic and treatment goals for subsequent outpatient management.

WHAT YOU NEED TO REMEMBER

- Numbness and tingling can be caused by a wide range of causes from the disabling but non–life-threatening, to the serious but chronic, to the acute and life-threatening.
- In the first 15 minutes, determine the acuity of onset, the rate of progression, and the presence of associated signs or symptoms, which would increase your concern for a life-threatening cause.
- Because sensation is subserved by various sensory modalities, each with specific tracts and nuclei and well-defined anatomic localization, your history and examination skills can be enormously valuable in localizing and diagnosing the patient's underlying condition.
- The sensory exam is largely subjective and strongly dependent on having a reliable and cooperative patient. The patient may be intentionally, or more often unintentionally, misleading with his or her reports of sensory findings. If the sensory exam is not internally consistent or is not consistent with other, more objective findings of the neurologic examination, be careful how much weight you place on the sensory examination.
- Evaluation is geared toward localization (sensory cortex, thalamus, brainstem, spinal cord, nerve root, nerve plexus, or peripheral nerve), because your differential diagnosis will be largely dependent on localization.
- Treatment is directed at both the underlying condition and the symptoms.
- Remember that your patient is lucky to have you working on his or her case. Most patients have only an overworked resident and/or distracted attending, and not a medical student with the time and motivation to truly understand the complexities of the presentation.

SUGGESTED READINGS

Buschbacher RM, Prahlow ND. *Manual of Nerve Conduction Studies.* 2nd Ed. New York: Demos Medical Publishing, 2005.

Dyck PJ, Thomas PK. *Peripheral Neuropathy.* 4th Ed. Philadelphia: WB Saunders, 2005.

Patten JP. *Neurological Differential Diagnosis.* 2nd Ed. New York: Springer, 1998.

Convulsions

THE PATIENT ENCOUNTER

A 56-year-old man presents to the emergency department following a convulsion that was accompanied by a decrease in his mental status. The convulsion lasted 3 minutes and occurred about an hour ago. The emergency department (ED) doctor now reports that the patient has not fully recovered his mental status and he is weak on his left side. His wife reports that he has never had a convulsion before. Over the last few weeks, he has had some incoordination on his left side.

OVERVIEW

Definition and Pathophysiology

Epileptic seizures are clinical phenomena (motor or sensory) that result from abnormally synchronized neuronal activity. *Epilepsy* is currently defined as two or more unprovoked seizures. Usually seizures that occur within a 24-hour period are counted as one seizure for the purposes of this definition. A "provoked seizure" is one that is caused by a clear trigger, but for which there is no ongoing predilection to epilepsy. So a seizure owing to encephalitis is provoked, whereas a patient who still has seizures several years after having had encephalitis has epilepsy.

Seizures are divided into two categories: partial and generalized. This is based on the electroencephalogram (EEG) findings more so than on the clinical findings. This division is the most important in terms of determining medical and surgical therapies. Partial seizures originate from one part of the brain (but may then spread), whereas generalized seizures, when recorded on an EEG, seem to originate from the entire brain at once.

- *Partial seizures*
  - Simple partial seizures (SPS):
    - Result in no change in mentation or level of consciousness
    - Include motor phenomena (unilateral, focal jerking), sensory phenomena (visual hallucination, olfactory hallucination), and/or psychic phenomena (déjà vu, feeling of rising in stomach like being on a roller coaster)

- Complex partial seizures (CPS):
  - Result in the presence of some change in mentation or level of consciousness (ranges from a mild change in higher cognitive abilities to complete unresponsiveness).
  - May be preceded by an aura (a simple partial seizure [SPS] that evolves into a CPS).
  - May present with no clear motor phenomena (i.e., staring spell).
  - May present with tonic motor activity (rigid, fixed extension or flexion).
  - May present with clonic motor activity (repetitious, rhythmic jerking).
  - Motor manifestations are often maximal on the side contralateral to the seizure focus.
  - Eye and head deviation is typically to the side opposite the seizure focus.
  - Automatisms are typically ipsilateral to the side of the seizure focus.
  - CPS may be followed by a postictal period of somnolence or confusion, lasting minutes to several hours.
  - Todd paralysis is a paresis in the postictal period and is typically contralateral to the seizure focus.
- Secondarily generalized CPS:
  - CPS may generalize—that is, spread to both sides of the brain. These seizures are also referred to as *secondarily generalized tonic-clonic seizures*, because they start with CPS semiology, then progress into a tonic ("stretching") phase and then a clonic ("jerking") phase.
  - The clinical appearance of the seizure at the onset (i.e., before the generalization) is the most important, because the early phase is what most helps localize the seizure onset.
- *Generalized seizures*
  - Primary generalized tonic-clonic seizures (1° GTC):
    - Typically, present as a symmetric tonic phase followed by a symmetric clonic phase.
    - Not preceded by auras.
    - Often have a postictal period.
    - Unlike secondarily generalized CPS, there are usually no focal features at the onset, and the tonic and clonic phases do not have asymmetries.
  - Myoclonic seizures:
    - Myoclonus is a single, lightning-fast jerk (often in arms/shoulders) or a shudder.
    - May have a cortical origin (epileptic) or subcortical origin (movement disorder).
  - Absence seizures:
    - Absence epilepsy is a specific syndrome that has an onset in childhood or adolescence. Although many staring spells are called "absence" (or by their old name, "petit mal"), most staring spells are, in fact, CPS.

- Absence seizures consist of several seconds of unresponsiveness. The patient is unaware that he or she has had one. A patient usually experiences tens to hundreds of them per day. There is no postictal period.
- Tonic and atonic seizures:
  - Tonic seizures consist of stiffening without a subsequent clonic phase. This often affects the axial musculature and may result in a fall. These typically occur in individuals with chronic neurologic disability.
  - Atonic seizures manifest as a sudden loss of body tone, and the patient "crumples" to the floor. The more mild manifestations may consist of a head drop. These typically occur in individuals with chronic neurologic disability.

Epidemiology

In the United States, seizure disorders are found in a bimodal age distribution targeting infants/adolescents as well as older folks (>65 years of age). There is no predilection for gender or ethnicity, but immigrants have a two-times higher prevalence of epilepsy because of childhood exposures to infectious organisms, such as toxoplasmosis, that affect the brain. Up to 1% of the population will experience at least a single seizure at some point in their lives, but in general, only 0.1% will develop an epilepsy disorder that requires treatment.

ACUTE MANAGEMENT AND WORKUP

There is long-standing debate about whether or not seizures cause permanent brain damage. The argument for shortening the length of the seizure is that permanent brain damage can result from prolonged hypoxia owing to poor respiration during the seizure. The argument against immediate intervention is that treating with short-acting anticonvulsants, such as benzodiazepines, will stop the seizures at the expense of suppressing mental status, which can lead to poor airway protection and aspiration pneumonia. A good general rule to apply to your patients is when you are confronted with the question of treating an actively seizing patient, consider intervention if the seizure lasts longer than usual for the patient or if the seizure lasts longer than 2 minutes.

The First 15 Minutes

Patients with seizures can present in two ways: actively seizing or postictal (already seized). The first 15 minutes of an actively seizing patient is spent in preventing further harm during the seizure and medically suppressing the seizure if it lasts longer than 2 minutes. In a patient who has stopped seizing, the first 15 minutes should be spent ruling out life-threatening conditions, such as intracranial hemorrhages, that can present with seizures. The acute management of both an actively seizing and a postictal patient is presented in the following section.

Initial Assessment

It may seem obvious, but initially, you have to determine whether your patient is actively seizing or has actually stopped seizing. Just because a patient is not shaking vigorously, it does not mean the seizure is over. Evidence of active seizing includes the following:

- Rhythmic shaking or tonic muscle contractions
- Eye deviation
- Altered mental status
- Stereotypic movements such as finger rubbing or lip smacking

It takes experience in dealing with seizure patients to know when a patient is seizing or when a patient is postictal. The most reliable way to tell is to get an EEG. However, it can be time-consuming and difficult to obtain an EEG and clinical acumen may be your only tool.

Acute Management of a Patient Who Is Actively Convulsing

If you decide the patient is actively convulsing when you initially meet him or her, you have four *immediate* responsibilities:

1. Make sure the patient's nurse and primary team are aware and get help.
2. Provide seizure first aid.
   - Move anything the patient may strike herself on, and make sure the patient is not in a position where she will fall.
   - Turn patient on her side so that she doesn't aspirate secretions or vomit.
   - Suction the patient's mouth (with appropriate assistance).
   - Provide oxygen.
3. Determine whether the patient is in status epilepticus (SE).
   - Although the most common definition of SE is a seizure that lasts 30 or more minutes (or multiple seizures without return to baseline between), abortive treatment begins after 2 minutes of seizing. Details about the types of treatment are discussed later in the chapter.
   - Get assistance from the primary team as well as the neurology house staff/attending and/or the critical care team.
4. Make careful observations of the convulsion.
   - Track how long the convulsion is lasting.
   - Check the patient's vital signs.
   - Assess responsiveness (provide auditory and tactile stimuli).
   - Assess memory (give the patient words to recall, and test after the convulsion has terminated).
   - Observe the patient's eyes: Are the patient's eyes open or closed? Are her eyes rolled back or deviated to one side?

- Observe the patient's face: Has her head deviated to one side? Is there jerking of her facial muscles?
- Observe the patient's limbs: Are they stretched out? Jerking? Flailing? Symmetric or asymmetric? Are there complex but purposeless movements (automatisms; e.g., picking at clothes or fumbling with items)?
- Note how the seizure evolves: What happens first; what happens later?
- Can you stop the jerking by applying pressure to a limb? (Do not apply pressure that is too hard, as you could cause dislocations.)
- What treatments have been given so far?
- Consider finger-stick blood glucose, electrolyte, and antiepileptic drug (AED) levels.
- If there is a question about whether the ongoing convulsions are actually epileptic, your resident may consider a stat EEG.

Acute Management of a Patient Who Is Not Actively Convulsing

In the acute phase, the most important question is whether the convulsion is merely a symptom of a more threatening condition.

When you first meet the patient, get a sense of her mental status and how "sick" she appears. That will help guide your suspicion for a malignant etiology for the convulsion. In the history, look for infectious and inflammatory conditions, neoplastic conditions, gastrointestinal (GI) and renal conditions, and recent toxic ingestions or withdrawal. Your neurologic review of systems should look for signs of hydrocephalus (e.g., in the case of tumor) and focal neurologic signs (e.g., indicating a mass lesion that may be epileptogenic).

The initial physical exam should evaluate vital signs—to look for fever, shock, cardiovascular instability, and hypertension. The general physical exam should address the possibility that a systemic disorder has caused the convulsions. In the neurologic exam, you should look at the patient's mental status to assess overall neurologic condition, and for focal deficits that might suggest a focal lesion that could also be epileptogenic.

Admission Criteria and Level of Care Criteria

Discharge from the emergency room is sometimes appropriate for patients who fit all of the following criteria:

1. Have convulsions that are well explained
2. Have convulsions that are not threatening
3. Are at a baseline level of functioning
4. Can be cared for safely at home
5. Have appropriate follow-up arranged for

For example, the ED may discharge a patient with long-standing epilepsy who has a cluster of seizures for which there is a good explanation and is addressed in the ED. A patient who clearly has a movement disorder but is otherwise well may have this addressed as an outpatient. On the other hand, a patient with recurrent psychogenic nonepileptic seizures may need an admission because he is not safe to go home.

When considering admission, the underlying etiology may dictate the disposition. For example, a patient with a brain tumor would likely go to the neurosurgery service, a patient with idiopathic seizures would likely go to neurology, and a patient with renal disease would likely go to internal medicine.

Unless there is *overwhelming* evidence that the patient has nonepileptic convulsions (e.g., psychogenic nonepileptic seizures), actively convulsing patients should be stabilized in an intensive care unit or an epilepsy monitoring unit. The treatment of *status epilepticus* involves medications that can suppress respiratory effort, and the patient must be in a setting where vital signs can be monitored continuously and intubation can be performed immediately.

Any patient who is having recurrent convulsions and who is not ill enough to be in an intensive care unit (ICU) should be placed in a situation where it will be apparent when he has convulsions. In various hospitals, this may be near the nurses' station, in a room with a sitter, or in an epilepsy monitoring unit.

Patients in whom there is a question about whether spells are epileptic or not can be admitted to an epilepsy monitoring unit under the following conditions: they are sufficiently stable that they do not need to be in the ICU, and their convulsions are occurring frequently enough that one is likely to be captured over the course of the admission.

When transferring your patient, make sure that the receiving nurses and team know the patient's course and what the patient's convulsions look like. Discuss the plan for management with your resident, and make sure that this information is communicated to the accepting team. Also communicate the results of any testing.

The First 24 Hours

Within the first 24 hours, the general goals of the evaluation are to determine the following:

1. The nature of the convulsions (i.e., differentiating among epileptic, other "organic," and psychogenic convulsions)
2. The cause of the convulsions
3. Whether the convulsions are adequately addressed at the moment

History

In determining the history of the present illness, including the nature of the patient's spells, it is important to assess the patient's overall history. As with all paroxysmal events in neurology, ask if this has ever happened before. The evaluation and management of a patient with long-standing epilepsy is quite different than that of a patient with a first convulsion. When taking a history, it is often critical to have a witness to the seizure because, in most cases, the patient is not aware of what is happening during the seizure.

In a patient who has an acute onset of new convulsions, the goals are to determine, first, the nature of the convulsions, and second, the cause of the convulsions. The previous section addressed the characteristics of seizures and of spells that can mimic seizures. Based on the information about seizures and seizure mimics noted previously, ask questions to determine which of those entities the patient's spells most seem like.

Your goals in evaluating a patient with a chief complaint of convulsions include obtaining information about the following:

1. *Preictal phase:*
   • Was there a premonition (a warning sign minutes to days before the seizure)?
   • Was there an aura (occurring seconds to a minute before the seizure)?
2. *Ictus:*
   • Ask:
     • What happens first
     • About what the patient experiences

CLINICAL PEARL

If the patient recalls and describes full body shaking, the event was likely to be nonepileptic because if both motor cortices are seizing, consciousness will almost always be compromised.

   • About the patient's responsiveness
   • About eye, head, and limb movements
   • How long the seizure lasted
3. *Postictal phase:*
   • Ask about any postictal somnolence or confusion.
   • Ask about Todd's paralysis.

Based on the answers to these questions, get an impression as to whether or not the convulsion was a seizure. If it was, then it is necessary to determine why the seizure occurred.

In a patient who presents with a chronic history of convulsions, the goals are slightly different. The first question to answer is why the patient has presented now. It could be for characterization of the spells. If this is the case, then the approach is the same as described previously. Given a longer history of the convulsions, you may ask a few additional questions:

1. What is the overall course of the convulsions? Are they getting better, getting worse, or staying the same?
2. In what context do the convulsions occur? Are they nocturnal? Diurnal? Catamenial (i.e., related to the menstrual cycle)?

3. What seems to trigger the convulsions? Fever or illness? Stress? Change in sleep schedule?

The answers to the questions above will provide you with good information that can help you to determine the differential diagnosis.

If a patient with known epilepsy presents with a cluster of seizures, then the first question to ask is if the seizures are those that the patient typically has. If the answer is "no," then you essentially have to start from scratch and work this up as a new issue. If, however, the seizures are typical, then the question is why they are occurring now. A common reason is that the medication is ineffective. This may be owing to noncompliance. Another common reason is that the administration of a non–antiepileptic medication has interfered with the metabolism of the antiepileptic medication. Also, non-neurologic illnesses (e.g., an intercurrent viral infection) and changes in the patient's sleep schedule can trigger seizures in a patient with epilepsy.

When interviewing a patient with epilepsy, the past medical history should include the following:

1. Risk factors for epilepsy
   - Febrile seizures as a child
   - Previous head trauma
   - Previous meningoencephalitis
   - Developmental disabilities
2. Previous test results
   - EEG results
   - EMU (epilepsy monitoring unit or video-EEG) results
   - MRI results (specifically looking for mesial temporal sclerosis)
   - PET (positron emission tomography) or SPECT (single photon emission computed tomography) scan results
3. All antiepileptic medications that have been tried in the past
   - Maximum doses
   - Efficacy
   - Side effects
   - Effective blood levels, if known

Physical Examination

You should perform a complete medical and neurologic physical examination, looking for any systemic illnesses that may have caused the seizures. The neurologic exam should look for focal lesions that may be epileptogenic (e.g., tumors or remote infarcts). The vast majority of patients with seizure disorder have normal physical exams when they are not seizing.

In your careful neurologic exam, look for the following findings:

- *Mental status.* Does the patient have momentary lapses of consciousness that are suggestive of partial complex seizures?

- *Cranial nerves.* Cranial nerves are generally normal in epileptic patients because brainstem lesions only rarely lead to seizures.
- *Motor exam.* Look for asymmetric weakness that suggests a focal lesion that may be a seizure focus in the brain.
- *Sensory exam.* Similar to the motor exam, the sensory exam should help you localize a cortical lesion that may be a seizure focus.
- *Reflexes.* Generally, reflexes are normal unless there is a focal lesion that affects the corticospinal tract in the brain or the subcortical white matter.
- *Coordination.* Cerebellar lesions are very rare causes of seizures, so the coordination exam should be normal.

In summary, patients with epilepsy who are not actively seizing and who are not immediately postictal generally have a normal exam unless there is a cortical or subcortical seizure focus that affects motor or sensory function.

Labs and Tests to Consider

Electroencephalograms (EEGs) are often ordered to assess patients with convulsions. They may provide you with the following information:

1. If the EEG is running at the exact time that the patient is having a seizure, then it can (almost) definitively tell whether the patient is having a seizure or not (this is the idea behind EMUs).
2. If you get an EEG immediately after a seizure, in the postictal period, the presence of focal findings may suggest that a focal seizure has occurred.
3. If you get an EEG at baseline between seizures (perhaps 48 hours after the last seizure), the presence of interictal discharges and focal findings may help you determine the nature of the seizure. Generalized interictal discharges are common in generalized epilepsies; focal interictal discharges (or focal slowing) are sometimes seen in patients with focal epilepsies. A normal EEG does not rule out that the patient has epilepsy.
4. An EEG can be used to assess for nonconvulsive status epilepticus. This is a situation in which the patient is no longer clearly convulsing physically but still has electrical seizure activity that manifests as change in mental status (sometimes with small twitching of the face and extremities).

Key Diagnostic Labs and Tests

Although the EEG is the test of choice for diagnosing the type of seizure disorders, other lab tests may be helpful if the EEG is suggestive of a common epileptic syndrome. For example, absence seizures cause very specific EEG patterns and can be diagnosed without any lab testing. In contrast, an EEG diagnostic of a nonspecific focal seizure may require a lumbar puncture and imaging to rule out a brain abscess that may be the focal seizure source. Table 6-1 lists the common labs that are obtained to help in the evaluation of seizure patients as well as the rationales for testing.

TABLE 6-1
Key Laboratory Tests and Rationales for Testing

Test	Rationale
Heme-8 with differential	Rule out (r/o) leukocytosis.
Basic metabolic panel	R/o evidence of metabolic dysfunction such as acute renal failure (ARF)/uremia, electrolyte imbalance such as hyponatremia.
Specific drug levels	E.g., phenytoin: If patient is on these medications, look at current level vs. patient's known therapeutic level.
Ethanol	R/o alcohol intoxication.
Urine toxicity	R/o toxic ingestion.
Urine pregnancy test	Because most AEDs are not so good for fetuses, you want to know before you start an AED in a pregnant woman.
Blood/urine cultures	If infection is suspected.

Imaging and Ancillary Testing
In the event that a focal lesion in the brain may be the cause of the seizure, the imaging and ancillary tests noted in Table 6-2 may prove useful in your workup. Another reason to obtain an MRI is consideration of surgical intervention for mesial temporal sclerosis.

Assessment
The assessment should comprise the following:

- Succinct summary sentence that describes the patient's age, which hand is the patient's dominant one, the relevant past medical history, and the overall course of convulsions
- Brief description of convulsions
- Differential diagnosis, including the type of seizure (if epileptic)

Differential Diagnosis
Several neurologic phenomena occur paroxysmally (i.e., in "attacks" or "spells"). Most of these fall into the categories of epileptic seizures, movement

TABLE 6-2
Key Imaging Tests and Rationales for Testing

Test	Rationale
Noncontrast head computed tomography (CT)	Rule out intracranial hemorrhage from stroke or subarachnoid hemorrhage, subdural hemorrhage from trauma, previous strokes, and hydrocephalus
Magnetic resonance imaging (MRI) of head	Looking for focal cortical pathology, masses, arteriovenous malformations (AVMs), cavernomas, evidence of hemosiderin, mesial temporal sclerosis

disorders, sleep disorders, cardiovascular disorders, and/or syncope, migraine, and psychogenic disorders.

1. Epileptic seizures
   - Seizures *are stereotypical* (i.e., each one looks similar to every other one). A patient may have several types of seizures, but each example within a certain type looks like the other.
   - *Seizures are resistant to outside stimuli.* A patient cannot be called out of an epileptic staring spell (unless the seizure was about to end by itself), and limb shaking caused by an epileptic seizure won't stop because someone holds it.
   - *Bilateral movements are almost always inconsistent with preserved consciousness.*
   - *Most seizures are 4 minutes or briefer in duration.* Longer spells are less likely to be seizures.
2. Movement disorders
   - Movement disorders represent a wide range of clinical entities, many with a pathophysiology that is presumed to be in the basal ganglia (whereas epileptic pathophysiology is primarily in the cortex).
   - Some movement disorders are paroxysmal and may be confused with epileptic seizures.
   - *Paroxysmal dyskinesias* involve attacks that last from seconds to many minutes and have a host of triggers. They are differentiated from seizures because consciousness and mentation are maintained, despite

bilateral body movements. The movements tend to be more ballistic rather than repetitive and rhythmic. Attacks can last significantly longer than most seizures tend to last.

- *Postanoxic myoclonus* occurs after a significant anoxic injury and can be difficult to differentiate from seizures. An EEG may be helpful in this case.

3. Sleep disorders
   - *Non-REM parasomnias* include somnambulism (sleepwalking), which could be mistaken for nocturnal seizures or the postictal period after a nocturnal seizure. It may take video-EEG monitoring to differentiate among these conditions.
   - *Narcolepsy* involves sleep attacks that could be confused with seizures. Cataplexy, insomnia, excessive daytime sleepiness, and sleep paralysis are other symptoms. Multiple sleep latency testing (in a sleep lab) is diagnostic.
   - *Cataplexy* is a symptom of narcolepsy and consists of a sudden loss of muscle tone following an emotional response with preserved awareness.

4. Cardiovascular disorders and/or syncope
   - Syncope results from decreased brain perfusion and can be associated with orthostatic hypotension and cardiac arrhythmias.
   - Convulsions can be seen following an abrupt loss of consciousness.
   - Testing may include orthostatic blood pressures, electrocardiogram (ECG), and at times, Holter monitoring and echocardiography.

5. Migraine
   - The sensory symptoms of migraine may be confused with seizures. However, whereas seizure symptoms tend to spread in a matter of seconds, the sensory phenomena of migraines spread over a period of minutes.

6. Psychogenic disorders
   - Psychogenic nonepileptic seizures (NES) were often referred to in the past as "pseudoseizures," although this term is considered pejorative.
   - Psychogenic disorders are similar to conversion disorders, in which the patient is typically unaware that the spells are psychogenic in nature and is not intentionally manufacturing them.
   - They may manifest as unresponsive episodes (i.e., the patient is aware of everything going on, but is unable to respond) or as convulsions.
   - The convulsions (or unresponsive spells) often go on for many minutes (longer than epileptic seizures typically last) and may not be followed by the postictal somnolence that would be typical for such a protracted seizure.
   - Alternatively, there may be evidence for preserved consciousness despite bilateral body movements.

- Although the semiology of the spell may lead an experienced clinician to suggest whether a convulsion is epileptic or not, a definitive diagnosis is made on the basis of video-EEG monitoring.
- Additional testing may include a psychiatric evaluation, though this is neither sensitive nor specific for NES (only 50% of NES patients have a diagnosable axis I disorder).

CLINICAL PEARL

A study has shown that patients who bring stuffed animals during their stay at the EEG monitoring unit are much more likely to have psychogenic seizures.

In the case of children and individuals with chronic neurologic disabilities, several other conditions can mimic seizures, including Sandifer syndrome, which is associated with gastroesophageal reflux and breath-holding spells.

Underlying Causes of Acute Seizures

Causes of acute seizures include the following:

- Infectious causes
  - Meningoencephalitis (especially herpes simplex encephalitis)
  - Abscess
- Neoplastic causes
  - Primary central nervous system (CNS) tumor
  - Metastases
- Cerebrovascular causes
  - Ischemic stroke
  - Bleeding
  - Arteriovenous malformation (AVM)
  - Subdural hematoma
  - Anoxia
- Toxic/metabolic causes
  - Illicit substances (e.g., cocaine)
  - Medications (e.g., bupropion, meperidine)
  - Withdrawal (e.g., ethanol—"delirium tremens")
  - Hypoglycemia and electrolyte abnormalities
  - Renal or hepatic disease
  - Hypertensive encephalopathy
  - Eclampsia
- Traumatic causes
  - Immediately after head trauma

Treatment

The treatment of nonepileptic convulsions depends on the nature of the convulsion:

- Movement disorders are usually treated with medications that target the dopaminergic system.
- Sleep disorders are often treated with the same dopaminergic therapies.
- Psychogenic disorders are treated with cognitive behavioral therapy, education, and occasional antidepressant medication as needed.
- In the case of epileptic seizures caused by an acute neurologic or systemic illness, treating that underlying illness is the standard of care. If seizures persist after treatment of the underlying illness, long-term antiepileptic therapy should be considered.

For treatment of epilepsy, the initial medical therapy is often selected by considering the significant side effects. For example, in a young married woman who is trying to get pregnant, valproic acid would be a poor choice because of teratogenic toxicity. Conversely, a man with comorbid migraines may benefit greatly from valproic acid's efficacy in preventing migraine headaches.

Choosing the "correct" first-line medication is subjective. Table 6-3 provides information about commonly used anticonvulsants.

EXTENDED INHOSPITAL MANAGEMENT

For patients who are admitted because they are unsafe to go home following the postictal period because they are either sleepy or sedated, the goal is to provide supportive care until the patients naturally recover, which is usually within 24 hours.

For patients who are admitted for workup of a new seizure disorder, extended hospital management may involve a workup that includes MRI, lumbar puncture, and possibly, a brain biopsy or tumor resection.

For patients who are admitted to the ICU with status epilepticus, extended hospital management involves complete suppression of epileptic activity for at least 24 hours, followed by slow weaning back to baseline. This may take days or longer and requires intensive monitoring and continuous EEG monitoring.

For patients who are admitted to an epilepsy monitoring unit either for consideration of surgery or to rule out a psychogenic cause of seizures, extended hospital management involves capturing a seizure event on the EEG and making treatment decisions based on those events.

DISPOSITION

Discharge Goals

The goals of discharge are the following:

- Identification of the nature of the convulsions
- Diagnosis and management of the cause of the convulsions

TABLE 6-3
Commonly Used Anticonvulsants

Drug	Indication	Notes
Carbamazepine (Tegretol)	Partial epilepsy	• Often first-line for partial epilepsy • Can cause Stevens-Johnson syndrome/toxic epidermal necrolysis • Can cause leukopenia and liver dysfunction • Can autoinduce metabolizing enzymes in liver
Oxcarbazepine (Trileptal)	Partial epilepsy	• Derivative of carbamazepine • Can cause hyponatremia • Can cause Stevens-Johnson syndrome/toxic epidermal necrolysis • Limited need for routine lab work
Phenytoin (Dilantin)	Partial epilepsy	• Can cause gingival hyperplasia, hirsutism, and bone demineralization • Not typically used in children chronically owing to fluctuating blood levels and narrow therapeutic window • Fosphenytoin can be given IV • Can cause Stevens-Johnson syndrome/toxic epidermal necrolysis
Valproate (Depakote)	Generalized or partial epilepsy	• Can lead to thrombocytopenia, pancreatitis, hyperammonemia, hair loss and weight gain, tremor • Particularly teratogenic • Can lead to liver failure in certain circumstances (young children, metabolic disease) • Can be given IV

(continued)

TABLE 6-3
Commonly Used Anticonvulsants (Continued)

Drug	Indication	Notes
Phenobarbital	Generalized or partial epilepsy	• Inexpensive • Very long half-life • Can lead to cognitive dulling, sedation and irritability • Can cause Stevens-Johnson syndrome/toxic epidermal necrolysis
Lamotrigine (Lamictal)	Generalized or partial epilepsy	• Can cause Stevens-Johnson syndrome/toxic epidermal necrolysis, especially if started at a high dose initially • Initial titration to effective dose must be slow • Dosing based on other meds patient is on (e.g., valproate or liver enzyme-inducing medications) • Less teratogenic than other AEDs • Blood levels change during and after pregnancy
Levetiracetam (Keppra)	Generalized or partial epilepsy	• Can cause irritability/mood changes • Can be given IV • No need for routine blood work
Topiramate (Topamax)	Generalized or partial epilepsy	• Can cause kidney stones, glaucoma (rarely), and cognitive dulling (common)
Ethosuximide (Zarontin)	Absence epilepsy	• Limited indication (specific for absence epilepsy) • Can cause stomach upset

TABLE 6-3
Commonly Used Anticonvulsants (Continued)

Drug	Indication	Notes
Zonisamide (Zonegran)	Generalized or partial epilepsy	• Can cause kidney stones • Long half-life • Sulfonamide
Pregabalin (Lyrica)	Partial epilepsy	• Can lead to weight gain and dizziness • Tablets only at this time

- Symptomatic management of the convulsions (e.g., medical treatment of the seizures)
- Ensuring that the patient has returned to baseline
- Education of the patient and family member regarding the following:
  - Seizure first aid
  - When to call the doctor (e.g., if there is an increase in seizure frequency or duration, or if there is a change in the seizure semiology)

Outpatient Care

Patients with convulsions need a plan for appropriate follow-up with an appropriate physician. In the case of seizures, this is a neurologist. Because seizures often recur, it is important that the patient and family have someone to contact in case another seizure occurs. Also, many seizure medications require laboratory monitoring, and this will be a part of ongoing care.

Seizures are also associated with a number of comorbid issues, including sleep problems, mood problems, and cognitive problems. All of these should be addressed as a part of ongoing care.

WHAT YOU NEED TO REMEMBER

- Convulsions can represent epileptic seizures, movement disorders, sleep phenomena, syncope, migraine, or psychogenic non-epileptic seizures.
- Epileptic seizures can be partial or generalized. Distinguishing between the two helps guide therapy.
- There are several causes of epileptic seizures. Some of these require immediate intervention.

SUGGESTED READINGS

AAN Guidelines on Epilepsy. Published yearly on AAN.com.

Bhardwaj A, Mirski MA, Ulatowski JA. *Handbook of Neurocritical Care.* 1st Ed. Totowa, NJ: Humana Press, 2004.

Engel J Jr, Pedley TA, Aicardi J, et al. *Epilepsy, A Comprehensive Textbook.* 2nd Ed. Philadelphia: Lippincott Williams & Wilkins, 2007.

Gait Disorders and Falls

A 77-year-old woman was brought in to the emergency department by ambulance after a fall. She is alert and oriented, but despite normal strength, she is unable to walk without a two-person assist and coaxing. She smells of urine. Her elderly husband says that over the past 2 years she has gradually lost her ability to walk easily around the house and rarely reaches the bathroom in time.

OVERVIEW

Definition and Pathophysiology

Gait disorders include all ailments that lead to problems walking, which, in turn, lead to falls. Gait disorders are generally categorized as neurologic and nonneurologic, but many patients present with multiple causes from both categories. Walking is a complex neurologic feat that requires many years of practice and coordination of many areas of the brain, spinal cord, peripheral nerves, muscles, and bones. A dysfunction of any one or more of these components may lead to a gait disorder.

Epidemiology

Gait disorders plague the elderly. According to the Einstein Aging Study, up to 35% of adults older than 70 years of age have a gait disorder (1). Men are somewhat more likely to develop a neurologic gait problem from strokes whereas women are more likely to have a nonneurologic gait disorder from orthopedic and arthritic problems. Institutionalization in a hospital or long-term facility or nursing home for any reason carries a threefold increase in the risk of developing a gait disorder.

ACUTE MANAGEMENT AND WORKUP

The goals of acute management in gait disorders and falls are twofold:

1. Workup for the cause of the gait disorder and/or fall
2. Workup for the consequences of the fall

The First 15 Minutes

The first 15 minutes in evaluating a patient with a typical long-standing gait disorder and falls is to rule out life-threatening consequences, mainly head trauma, as a result of the fall. Keep in mind that head trauma in the elderly can easily cause subdural hematomas that may take hours or days to present with signs and symptoms.

In a patient who was previously healthy and who suddenly developed gait abnormalities and falls, your first 15 minutes should be spent assessing for life-threatening conditions of acute causes of gait disorders, such as strokes, hemorrhages, and multiple sclerosis.

Initial Assessment

The initial assessment of patients with gait and balance disorders should focus on the most common urgent consequence of these disorders: falls. The case study patient is alert and oriented, so it is likely that her ABCs (airway, breathing, and circulation) are intact, but could she have an injury from the fall that might cause her to become unstable?

1. *Check the patient's vital signs.* Check the vital signs at arrival and examine the patient thoroughly until you feel confident there are no major injuries from the fall, such as bleeding in the hip or head.
2. *Arrange for rapid imaging to look for emergent signs.* Obtain and review appropriate imaging to assess for possible emergent issues:
   • Head CT. This should be obtained for all elderly patients after a fall; look for epidural, subdural, or parenchymal hemorrhage, and for fracture of the skull.
   • Spinal CT. Arrange for a spinal CT to assess for fracture if there is spine tenderness or radiating pain that suggests a spinal injury.
   • X-rays. Arrange for plain films to evaluate possible fractures of the neck, hips, pelvis, and long bones; in the case of our patient, the left hip should be x-rayed.
   • Pelvic CT. Consider a CT scan of the pelvic region to evaluate for hemorrhage if vital signs become unstable, hip pain continues to increase, or bruising continues to expand.
3. *Arrange for appropriate laboratory tests.* Send urine for analysis and culture, and blood for a complete blood count and complete metabolic panel to confirm that no metabolic abnormalities contributed to the fall.

Admission Criteria and Level of Care Criteria

Most patients with gait disorders are seen in the outpatient clinic. Frequently, however, elderly patients are brought to the emergency room after a relatively minor fall that has produced no significant injuries. By interviewing the patient and family, you may find that the fall represents the culmination of a long, slow deterioration in mobility. If the patient has been living alone, she may have gradually lost the ability to manage her home and perform self-care. If the patient lives with relatives, he may arrive at the emergency room after a trivial fall because his relatives are at the end of their ability to cope with severe mobility impairment and the associated incontinence.

Even if the blood tests are normal and you identify no significant injuries, you may need to admit the patient with progressive impairment of mobility for further workup, assessment by physical therapy, rehabilitation, and evaluation of the patient's living situation by a social worker.

You can admit a cooperative patient with progressive mobility impairment to a standard medical floor, but make certain to request fall precautions so that the nurses are aware of the patient's fall risk.

The First 24 Hours

Once your patient is comfortably stable and admitted to the hospital for workup and treatment, the first 24 hours should be designed to complete a thorough workup tailored to your patient's specific situation. The history and physical are important for helping you plan the lab testing and imaging that may be necessary to help you make the diagnosis.

History

A thorough history can provide important clues to the cause of a progressive gait disorder. Even if the patient has no cognitive impairment, you should interview family members or others who have observed your patient over the past few years. A patient may minimize her own impairment, particularly if she is worried she might be moved into a nursing home. In addition, a patient might not notice the first subtle changes associated with Parkinson disease, spinal stenosis, or adult hydrocephalus, but the patient's family members often do.

The items that follow include the questions you will need to ask, the actions you will need to take, and patient care aspects you will need to consider when you gather the patient's history.

- *History of mobility impairment.* Questions to ask both the patient and family include the following:
  1. How long ago did she last walk normally, without an assistive device? This question will help you gauge the duration and progression of symptoms. Gait disorders can develop quickly in the case of a cerebellar stroke, for example, or slowly, over years, in the case of Parkinson's disease.
  2. Has she fallen before? What were the circumstances? Did she go to the emergency room for other falls? Get an idea of the severity

of the condition. Frequent falls and emergency room visits suggest a severe condition and may prompt an admission for a safety evaluation.

3. Which assistive devices does she use in the home, for short trips, and for longer excursions? The use of a cane suggests mild impairment, whereas use of a wheelchair suggests more progressive impairment. If she doesn't use an assistive device, does she instead touch the furniture and walls for added balance while walking around the house?

4. Does walking cause pain? If so, where? How long has she experienced this pain? Does the pain stop when she stops walking?

5. Does walking cause shortness of breath? If so, does she have known lung or heart disease? If the answer is yes to shortness of breath, but she has not been evaluated for lung or heart disease, consider a detour to cardiac and pulmonary testing.

6. Is she most likely to fall in dim light or in the shower? Both suggest loss of proprioception, which is often associated with peripheral neuropathy from diabetes or heavy alcohol use.

7. Are her movements slow? Has she developed a tremor? Has her facial expression become masked? These signs are suggestive of Parkinson disease and related disorders.

8. Does she ever start speeding up when she's walking and lose control of her ability to stop? This is referred to as *festination*, which is suggestive of Parkinson disease and related disorders, and rarely, adult hydrocephalus.

- *History of Related Issues.*
  1. Has the family noticed changes in affect or cognition over the past several years? This is suggestive of a progressive dementia, which may be associated with mobility impairment. Even Parkinson's disease may cause an alteration of affect or cognition.
  2. Has the patient experienced any urinary urgency or incontinence? Urinary urgency is an early sign of adult hydrocephalus. Most patients with mobility impairment from any cause will eventually have episodes of incontinence because of inability to reach a toilet.

- *Past Medical History.* Record all of the patient's history, but make special note of knee or hip surgery, arthritis, back surgery, and pulmonary or cardiac disease.

- *Medications.* Review all medications the patient is taking, especially those that are new or recently dose adjusted. Medications particularly known for impairing the balance and gait of elderly patients include benzodiazepines, sleeping aids, opiates, and anticholinergics (e.g., Benadryl). Elderly patients may also be impaired by the use of multiple blood pressure medications or by an enormous number of diverse medications collectively prescribed over many years.

- *Social History.* Find out who currently lives with or assists your mobility-impaired patient in activities of daily living. If you suspect the family has reached a limit in caretaking ability, request a social worker consult. Find out if there is a history of heavy alcohol use and if there is current alcohol use.

> ### CLINICAL PEARL
>
> *Fewer than 50% of elderly alcoholics are diagnosed because the signs are masked by denial and apparent good health. Is your patient obtaining adequate nutrition? Deficiencies in B12, vitamin E, or other nutrients may lead to treatable gait impairment.*

Physical Examination

Perform a complete general and neurologic exam. Refer to Chapter 1, Localization and the Neurologic Exam, for details on performing a neurologic examination.

Make sure to perform these key parts of the exam:

- *Neck.* Check the patient's range of motion. Does movement of the neck cause pain that suggests radiculopathy? Limited movement of the neck suggests arthritis and possible cervical stenosis.
- *Mental status.* Perform Mini Mental Status Examination (MMSE) and other bedside tests of cognition. (Advancing dementia is often associated with balance and gait impairment.)
- *Spine.* Palpate the spine from neck to sacrum. Is there any tenderness or scoliosis? Does a straight-leg raise cause pain? This finding suggests radiculopathy or stenosis in the lumbosacral region.
- *Cranial nerves.* Look for limited movement of the facial muscles associated with Parkinson's disease, and abnormalities of eye movements associated with progressive supranuclear palsy and progressive dementias. Ptosis, abnormalities of eye movements, and impaired swallow may also lead you toward a workup for myasthenia gravis, which may first present in older patients.
- *Motor function.* Gait impairment can occur in patients with or without weakness. Carefully document the strength of the patient's legs and arms. A strong patient who cannot walk may be impaired by pain, loss of proprioception, ataxia caused by disorders of the cerebellum or inner ear, or disruption of cerebral connections owing to adult hydrocephalus or subcortical small vessel disease. Check also for patterns of weakness, which suggest cervical or lumbar stenosis, or radiculopathy. Muscle tone

is helpful in localizing lesions as well. Increased tone is suggestive of an upper motor neuron problem whereas decreased tone is suggestive of lower motor neuron dysfunction. Cogwheel rigidity is seen in disorders of the basal ganglia such as Parkinson's disease.

- *Sensory function.* Check the patient's toes and feet for reduced sensation to fine touch, pinprick, vibrating tuning fork, and proprioception. Gently walk the point of a new safety pin up each foot and leg to evaluate for length-dependent neuropathy.
- *Reflexes.* Check reflexes and the Babinski reflex. Increased reflexes and clonus at the ankles suggest cervical or thoracic myelopathy. Decreased or absent lower limb reflexes suggest lumbar myelopathy.
- *Gait.* Thoroughly evaluate all aspects of the patient's mobility. You may find a standardized test helpful, such as the Tinetti Assessment Tool (2), from which the following checklist is adapted:
  - Impaired bed mobility, which includes an inability to pull oneself to a sitting position
  - Impaired ability to sit up without a backrest
  - Impaired ability to stand up from a chair without assistance
  - Impaired ability to stand without an assistive device
  - Wide-based stance or gait
  - Ataxic movements (lurching)
  - Short steps
  - Foot dragging
  - Slow gait
  - Difficulty with turns
  - Positive Romberg test (suggests proprioceptive difficulties)
  - Inability to stand on one foot (check for weakness and imbalance)
  - Inability to walk in tandem (i.e., to place one foot right in front of the other foot)
  - Pain with walking
  - Shortness of breath that is induced by walking
  - A rapid onset of fatigue
- *Skin.* Check for skin breakdown on the buttocks and groin.

Labs and Tests to Consider

Based on your history and physical exam, consider ordering labs and imaging studies that will help you identify or confirm the cause of the gait disorder. Much of the workup is similar to other neurologic disorders, but there are a few tests that are unique to gait disorders.

Key Diagnostic Labs and Tests

One key diagnostic laboratory value is the patient's vitamin B12 level. Vitamin B12 deficiency can present with dorsal column dysfunction that leads to falls, especially in the dark.

> ### CLINICAL PEARL
>
> *To reliably rule out vitamin B12 deficiency, be sure to send for a methylmalonic acid (MMA) level that provides the best indication of long-standing vitamin B12 deficiency. The second test important in gait disorders is the opening pressure from a spinal tap in ruling out normal-pressure hydrocephalus (NPH). In addition to measuring opening pressure, the diagnosis of NPH is confirmed if the gait improves within an hour of the tap.*

Table 7-1 lists the tests and rationales for the workup of gait disorders.

Imaging and Ancillary Testing

The goal of imaging patients with gait disorders is to rule out a focal lesion that affects either the sensory or motor pathways important in walking. As mentioned in the introduction of this chapter, walking is a complex task that involves many different parts of the central and peripheral nervous systems. A lesion in any part may lead to a gait disorder.

One unique imaging test for diagnosing NPH, a common cause of gait problems, is the sagittal T1 sequence of the MRI. In this view, you may be able to appreciate bowing of the corpus callosum, which is suggestive of increased ventricular pressure in NPH. Table 7-2 lists the common imaging tests and rationales for a broad workup of gait disorders.

Assessment

As with any neurologic workup, there are three components that compose your assessment:

- *A succinct, summary sentence that includes the most important aspects of the history, physical exam, and tests.* For example, "A 77-year-old woman presents with 2 years of gradually progressive gait impairment and urinary incontinence in the context of normal strength and intact cognition."
- *Localization.* The history and physical exam alone frequently identify the regional location of the lesion, but a more definitive answer may be revealed by MRI or other testing modalities.
- *Differential diagnosis.* Most elderly patients have multiple contributing causes of gait impairment and thus multiple sites of localization; for example, a patient may have generalized arthritis, an injured knee, moderate small vessel disease, a remote cerebellar stroke, and B12 deficiency. Obviously, correcting one problem will improve only the proportion of disability owing to that particular problem. Try to discern which contributing causes are most responsible for impairment and start treatment

TABLE 7-1
Key Laboratory Tests and Rationales for Testing

Test	Rationale
Heme-8 w/diff, CMP, UA	Rule out infection or metabolic dysfunction.
Specific levels of medications	For example, check phenytoin and lithium levels as these medications are known to affect gait.
TSH	Abnormal thyroid levels can cause weakness.
B12, methylmalonic acid	A deficiency can cause impairment of gait owing to demyelination of the posterior columns plus peripheral neuropathy.
Other B complex vitamins and vitamin E	Suspicion of nutritional compromise or a history of GI surgery or disease.
Lumbar puncture	If imaging suggests hydrocephalus, evaluate patient with validated gait tools (for example, Timed Up and Go and Tinetti Assessment Tool) before and 30 minutes after draining 30–50 mL of CSF. Send CSF for basic labs and VDRL to rule out neurosyphilis.

CMP, cytidine monophosphate; UA, urinalysis; TSH, thyroid-stimulating hormone; GI, gastrointestinal; CSF, cerebrospinal fluid; VDRL, Venereal Disease Research Laboratories [test].

for those problems first. A list of causes by localization is provided in Table 7-3.

Treatment

Determine the most likely causes for gait and balance impairment, perform additional tests to confirm the cause(s), and treat whichever contributing factors are treatable. Most patients will need referrals to an outpatient clinic for full evaluation (for example, orthopedic surgeon for possible knee replacement, neurologist to follow response to medications for suspected

TABLE 7-2
Key Imaging Tests and Rationales for Testing

Test	Rationale
Noncontrast head computed tomography (CT)	Rule out subdural hematoma and hydrocephalus
Magnetic resonance imaging (MRI) of brain	Rule out extensive small vessel disease on FLAIR sequence, multiple lacunar strokes, neoplasm, multiple sclerosis, cerebellar degeneration or stroke; sagittal T1 sequence to rule out NPH
MRI of cervical/thoracic/lumbar spine	Rule out cervical or thoracic myelopathy or radiculopathy, as well as degenerative disc disease
Electromyogram/nerve Conduction study (EMG/NCS)	Rule out neuropathy, radiculopathy, and plexopathy
Electroencephalogram (EEG)	If the history suggests intermittent gait impairment/falls, which are concerning for seizure activity

FLAIR, fluid-attenuated inversion recovery; NPH, normal-pressure hydrocephalus; EMG/NCS, electromyogram/nerve conduction study; EEG, electroencephalogram.

Parkinson's disease). Go through each patient's list of medications carefully to see if any might be contributing to imbalance. If the medication list is long, discuss it with the patient's primary doctor to determine whether any medications can be eliminated. Table 7-4 lists the standard care for patients with gait disorders.

EXTENDED INHOSPITAL MANAGEMENT

All patients admitted for balance and gait impairment should be evaluated by a physical therapist and an occupational therapist. Physical therapists focus on the mechanical aspects of standing and walking and devise ways to improve strength and mobility. Occupational therapists focus on improving the patient's ability to perform activities of daily living that may be limited by his or her gait impairment. Elderly patients presenting with long-standing

TABLE 7-3
Causes of Chronic Gait Impairment by Localization

System	Localization	Etiology
Neurologic	Brain	Multiple small infarcts, periventricular small vessel disease, neoplasm, adult hydrocephalus, demyelinating disease, degenerative dementias, Parkinson's disease, essential tremor, subdural hematoma, cerebellar degeneration, amyotrophic lateral sclerosis (ALS)
	Spine/root	Cervical stenosis, lumbar stenosis, disc herniation, neoplasm, degenerative disease, venous plexus malformation, vitamin deficiencies
	Peripheral nerves	Neuropathy, vestibular dysfunction, myopathies, myasthenia gravis
Orthopedic	Lower extremities	Hip, knee, or foot problems
Rheumatologic	Systemic	Arthritis, autoimmune diseases

progressive impairment will likely require transfer to a rehabilitation facility. A social worker should be involved to help determine whether a discussion regarding long-term placement or additional home resources, such as a hospital bed, bedside commode, and/or wheelchair, would be helpful.

DISPOSITION
Discharge Goals
The goals of discharge are the following:

- Specific plans to continue the outpatient workup of any potentially treatable disorders that contribute to the patient's gait and balance impairment
- Specific plans to provide the patient and family with improved resources to cope with the gait and balance impairment

TABLE 7-4
Treatment of Gait Disorders by Etiology

Etiology	Treatment
Stroke, vascular disease	Modification of stroke risk factors to prevent another stroke and physical therapy to improve chances of recovery
Demyelinating disease	Immunosuppression
Normal pressure hydrocephalus	CSF shunting
Neoplasm	Neurosurgical and oncologic consultation
Parkinson's disease	Dopaminergic agents
Essential tremor	Beta-blocker or low-dose benzodiazepines
Subdural hematoma	Surgical drainage vs. close observation
Neurodegenerative diseases	Physical therapy to maximize remaining function
Cervical stenosis, radiculopathy	Neurosurgical consultation and physical therapy
Vitamin deficiencies	Repletion of vitamins
Peripheral neuropathy	Control of underlying disease that led to peripheral neuropathy plus symptomatic treatment of pain as needed to improve function
Orthopedic abnormalities	Orthopedic consultation and physical therapy
Rheumatologic abnormalities	Rheumatology consultation and physical therapy

Outpatient Care

As mentioned previously, most gait disorders are managed in the outpatient clinic. Depending on the specific cause, your patient may require a specialist such as a movement disorder expert (for example, for Parkinson's disease), a stroke expert, or a neurosurgeon. A follow-up appointment should also be arranged to care for the consequences (if any) of the fall.

WHAT YOU NEED TO REMEMBER

- There are myriad causes of gait and balance impairment, particularly in elderly patients, and most patients have more than one contributing factor.
- Patients are often brought to the hospital following a long, progressive deterioration in mobility, when the family is no longer capable of caring for the patient at home.
- Some patients will be able to return home if one or more treatable causes of impairment are addressed. Most will require physical therapy and additional adaptive resources or homecare helpers.
- Some patients may need to move to long-term care facilities because of severe mobility impairment and lack of capable caregivers.

REFERENCES

1. Verghese J, LeValley A, Hall CB, et al. Epidemiology of gait disorders in community-residing older adults. *J Am Geriatr Soc* 2005;54(2):255–261.
2. Tinetti ME. Performance-oriented assessment of mobility problems in elderly patients. *J Am Geriatr Soc* 1986;34(2):119–126.

SUGGESTED READINGS

Ashton-Miller J, Hausdorff JM, Alexander NB. *Gait Disorders: Evaluation and Management.* 1st Ed. London, UK: Informa Healthcare, 2005.
Masdeu JC, Sudarsky L, Wolfson L. *Gait Disorders of Aging: Falls and Therapeutic Strategies.* Philadelphia: Lippincott-Raven Publishers, 1997.
Ruzicka E, Hallett M, Jankovic J. *Advances in Neurology, Vol. 87: Gait Disorders.* Lippincott Williams & Wilkins, 2001.

Dizziness

THE PATIENT ENCOUNTER

A 55-year-old accountant woke up this morning feeling dizzy. He says it feels like the room is spinning around him in a counterclockwise direction. The only way to make it stop is to lie very still. The dizziness causes nausea, and he has vomited a couple of times this morning. He has no other complaints such as weakness, sensory changes, or tinnitus.

OVERVIEW

Definition and Pathophysiology

Patients who come to the emergency department (ED) with dizziness often use *dizziness* to mean various sensations. Physicians need to help patients refine exactly what they mean by dizziness. Neurologists define "dizziness" as *either*:

- **Vertigo.** An inappropriate sense of motion of either oneself or one's environment. Patients often report feeling the room spin or that they are spinning within the room.
- **Light-headedness.** A sense of reduced awareness of the environment without actual loss of consciousness, also called *faintness* and *giddiness*. *Presyncope* is the feeling of the world closing in on one, a sense of "vision closing in," like in a tunnel, or an impending loss of consciousness, just before experiencing syncope.

True vertigo always involves the inner ear, the eighth cranial nerve, the brainstem, or the deep cerebellum. Vertigo is considered peripheral when the cause is localized to the inner ear or the eighth cranial nerve, and is considered central when the cause is localized to the brainstem or the deep cerebellum.

In contrast, light-headedness can be broadly placed into four categories:

- **Neurologic.** The most concerning cause of neurologic light-headedness is hypoperfusion to the brainstem. The brainstem is supplied primarily by the vertebral arteries and basilar artery but can receive collateral circulation from the carotid arteries via the circle of Willis. A decrease in blood flow in any of these arteries, but especially the basilar, can cause light-headedness. Other neurologic causes of nonvertiginous dizziness or light-headedness include autonomic neuropathy and basal ganglia or cerebellar disturbances, which lead to feelings of imbalance and unsteadiness.

- **General Medical.** The primary general medical complications include hypotension, especially orthostatic, and hypoglycemia and other metabolic/toxic disturbances, thiamine (B1) deficiency, diabetes, hypothyroidism arrhythmias, myocardial infarction and aortic dissection.
- **Psychiatric.** The primary psychiatric complaints include anxiety (with hyperventilation), phobias, and somatoform disturbances.
- **Medications.** Medications that may cause "dizziness," and many other symptoms, include antiepileptics, sedatives, hypnotics, and antianxiety agents.

Epidemiology

Dizziness is a common complaint, accounting for about 2.5% of all complaints to a primary care physician's office. In general, the incidence increases with age. Neurologic causes of dizziness are responsible for <10% of cases, but neurologists are often the first consultants referred by generalists and ER physicians. Otologic causes of dizziness are by far the most common.

ACUTE MANAGEMENT AND WORKUP

The initial part of the evaluation is to use the history of the present illness to help you determine if the complaint of dizziness is vertigo or lightheadedness. If it is vertigo, next try to localize the problem to a peripheral or central cause. If the history suggests light-headedness, the scope is broadened and includes neurologic and nonneurologic workups.

The First 15 Minutes

Central causes of dizziness can be life-threatening, which makes determining the origin of vertigo or light-headedness essential. An acute onset of either vertigo or light-headedness that localizes to the brainstem or cerebral circulation should be treated as a neurologic emergency!

Initial Assessment

The initial assessment of a patient with dizziness should focus on the brainstem and cerebellum because dysfunction in these areas may imply further impending harm to a part of the brain that is vital for life. A stroke in the circulation around the brainstem that initially causes dizziness may get worse quickly and may lead to a complete brainstem infarct and death. Similarly, a hemorrhage in the deep cerebellum that presents as vertigo may swell and lead to compression of the brainstem and death. Cerebellar tumors, demyelination of the brainstem in multiple sclerosis, and infections such as meningitis or encephalitis can all present with dizziness that rapidly worsen to coma or death. Any components of the history, the physical, or imaging that suggest localization to the brainstem or cerebellum should prompt a full neurologic workup.

TABLE 8-1
Components That Suggest Localization to the Brainstem or Cerebellum

History	• Complaint of acute neck pain prior to onset (think: vertebral dissection) • Complaint of double vision • Complaint of weakness in face or "face looks twisted" and *contralateral* body • Complaint of sensory change in the face and *contralateral* body
Physical	• Cranial nerve abnormality(ies) • Weakness in the face and *contralateral* body • Sensory changes in the face and *contralateral* body • Direction-changing nystagmus
Imaging	• Any abnormality in the brainstem or cerebellum

Components of the history, physical exam, or imaging that suggest a localization to the brainstem or cerebellum are listed in Table 8-1.

Admission Criteria and Level of Care Criteria

Considerations for admission include the following:

• Any patient *suspected* of having a posterior circulation stroke or transient ischemic attack (TIA) of any cause must be admitted to a stroke unit if available; otherwise, the patient should be admitted at least to an intermediate care floor as he or she is at risk for worsening or for an extension of the infarct.
• Any patient with vertigo severe enough that he or she is deemed unable to keep down food, water, or medications
• Any patient with a newly diagnosed mass lesion, or an enlarging previously known mass
• Any patient with a new imaging abnormality in the brainstem or cerebellum
• Any patient with a suspected neurologic cause of dizziness

In general, patients with a peripheral cause of vertigo, such as inflammation of the eighth cranial nerve (vestibular neuritis), can be treated as an outpatient. However, it is better to err on the side of caution and admit a patient to the hospital if a central lesion cannot be reliably ruled out.

The First 24 Hours

In the first 24 hours of admission, the goal is to obtain all testing needed to help make the diagnosis and to begin treatment if possible.

History

In any patient with dizziness, whether light-headedness or vertigo, you should address the following points in the history of the present illness:

- *Medications.* Go over the medication list. Have any new medications been started recently? Usual offenders include anticonvulsants, sedatives, antidepressants, hypnotics, and antihypertensives.
- *History of mobility impairment.* Ask if the symptoms are constant or are present only with certain maneuvers. Vertigo triggered by horizontal movements of the head point to dysfunction of the semicircular canals. Light-headedness triggered by standing up suggests cerebral hypoperfusion.
- *History of related issues.*
  - ***Essential Point:*** Are there associated symptoms, such as diplopia, dysphagia, or dysarthria, that point to a brainstem cause, including vertebral-basilar insufficiency?
  - Determine if there is a history of recent viral infections (which suggest a harbinger of vestibular neuritis), of head trauma (causing benign paroxysmal positional vertigo [BPPV]), or of a nutritional deficiency (B1 deficiency).
  - Ask about vascular risk factors, including diabetes, hypertension, hyperlipidemia, previous myocardial infarction or strokes, and a family history.
- *Time course of events.* Ask about the time course of events. Did the dizziness start acutely, or was it intermittent or chronic? The time course will help you determine the cause.

Physical Examination

Following a complete general and neurologic exam, consider the following components in evaluating a patient with dizziness:

- *Vital signs.* Check the patient's blood pressure, both lying down and standing up. Orthostatic patients will feel light-headed when standing or sitting up.
- *General exam.* Is the patient in distress? Is the patient vomiting? Or is he or she comfortable and only complains when moved?

CLINICAL PEARL

Intense vertigo suggests a peripheral cause (i.e., inner ear or eighth cranial nerve), whereas a lower-intensity and constant vertigo suggests a central origin, but there are frequent exceptions.

- *Cardiac function*. Occasionally, myocardial infarction and aortic dissection may present with dizziness. Check for abnormal rhythms and assess for cardiogenic failure by auscultating for pulmonary edema for left-sided failure, and measure jugular venous pressure for right-sided failure.
- *Neurologic function*.
  - Mental status. Is the patient alert and oriented? Posterior fossa (e.g., cerebellar hemorrhages that compress the brainstem) and posterior circulation problems (e.g., basilar thrombosis) can cause a decreased or an altered mental status. Keep in mind that by the time you evaluate the patient, the emergency room staff might have given an antiemetic, which may cause drowsiness.
  - Cranial nerves. Consider the following:
    I: Rarely provides meaningful information, unless you suspect facial trauma, which can cause anosmia owing to shearing of the olfactory nerve.
    II: Look for papilledema, as a sign of increased intracranial pressure as might be seen in brain masses that occupy large spaces.
    II, IV, VI: This is where you must invest a significant amount of time during the physical exam. Look for any nystagmus, and try to define it:
    - Is it present during straight-ahead fixation or on eccentric gaze? How intense is it? A few beats of nystagmus on a far eccentric gaze may be normal.
    - Is it vertical, torsional, or horizontal? Is it induced by any maneuvers? Pure vertical nystagmus almost always suggests a central cause. When performing the Dix-Hallpike maneuver, vertigo and nystagmus often appear after a 5- to 15-second delay (Fig. 8-1).
    - Are there any limitations of extraocular motion? This generally indicates a brainstem lesion, which, when acute, should make you suspicious of a stroke. Wernicke's encephalopathy (B1 deficiency) must always be considered if eye movements are restricted in all directions (known as ophthalmoplegia).
    V: Hemisensory loss on the face paired with contralateral sensory loss is a crossed finding that almost always localizes to the brainstem.
    VII: Determine if there is facial asymmetry. Facial asymmetry at rest, with a smile or while talking or chewing, should be further characterized as central or peripheral. A peripheral seventh cranial nerve lesion causes weakness of an entire half of the face, including the brow, cheek, and lips. This finding can be elicited by asking the patient to close his or her eyes tightly against resistance. If you are easily able to open the eye, the patient is weak. The same is true of the lips. A peripheral seventh can be caused by either dysfunction of the cranial nerve itself (i.e., Bell palsy) or the seventh cranial nerve nucleus within the brainstem.

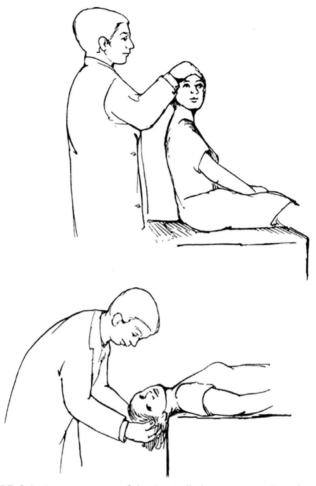

FIGURE 8-1: Demonstration of the Dix-Hallpike maneuver. First, have the patient sit on the edge of the bed and turn her head to one side. Quickly and safely, lay the patient down with her head just below the level of the bed while still turned. Watch for torsional nystagmus in the direction of the affected ear within 15 seconds. If none, repeat the maneuver with the patient's head facing the opposite direction.

In contrast, a central seventh is caused by an asymmetric cortical or subcortical lesion. Recall that the seventh cranial nerve nucleus that innervates the upper face receives input from both cortices. Thus, an asymmetric cortical or subcortical lesion will hardly affect the contralateral upper face because the seventh cranial nerve nucleus is receiving inputs from the ipsilateral cortex as well. However, the part of the seventh cranial nerve nucleus that innervates the lower face receives input from only the contralateral cortex. Thus, if the neurons or their tracts that run from the cerebral cortex of the inferior frontal lobe, which innervates the face, are damaged, the contralateral lower face will lose innervation and will be weak compared to the intact side of the face.

VIII: The evaluation of this nerve's function is very important in a dizzy/vertiginous patient. Detecting a loss of hearing may suggest a lateralizing peripheral lesion. Strokes involving the labyrinthine artery (or its usual source, the anterior inferior cerebellar artery, AICA) can also present with acute decreased hearing with other signs of a loss of labyrinthine function.

IX, X, XII: Make sure the palate is elevated and the patient's tongue is midline to help exclude a brainstem lesion.

- Motor strength. Asymmetry in strength and weakness may point to a cerebrovascular event. Are the symptoms contralateral from any cranial nerve deficits? This "crossed finding" localizes the lesion to the brainstem.
- Sensation. Is there a crossed sensory change between the face and the body? If so, consider a brainstem lesion.
- Coordination. Cerebellar lesions will cause dysmetria ipsilateral to the lesion, which means that a right cerebellar stroke will cause dysmetria of the right arm and leg.
- Gait. Difficulty walking, with falling to one side, may be an early sign of cerebellar dysfunction.

Labs and Tests to Consider

The basic laboratory testing listed in Table 8-2 helps rule out many of the nonneurologic systemic illnesses that causes dizziness. Many common nonneurologic conditions that present with dizziness, such as urinary tract infections and myocardial infarctions, can be quickly assessed by laboratory testing. Also included in Table 8-2 are the key serologic and cerebrospinal fluid tests that can be considered on a comprehensive dizziness workup.

Key Diagnostic Labs and Tests

Table 8-2 lists the tests and rationales for the workup of dizziness.

Imaging and Ancillary Testing

MRI is the ideal imaging modality for patients presenting with dizziness because CT scan images cannot penetrate the thick posterior skull well enough to visualize the brainstem and cerebellum at a high resolution. Nevertheless, as listed in Table 8-3, a CT scan should be obtained first because it is quick and rules out a hemorrhagic emergency. An MRI should be

TABLE 8-2
Key Diagnostic Labs to Work up Dizziness

Test	Rationale
CBC with differential	Leukocytosis, anemia indicates systemic illness
Complete metabolic panel	Hypoglycemia/hyperglycemia
Cardiac enzymes	Rule out MI
Urinalysis	Rule out UTI
Blood cultures	Bacteremia
Antiepileptic drugs levels	Drug intoxication
HIV test	At-risk populations that may present with opportunistic infections such as toxoplasmosis
Lumbar puncture; only after ruling out mass effect	When appropriate: concern for infectious masses
	Neurosyphilis, toxoplasmosis, CNS lymphoma
ECG	Are they in sinus rhythm? Any other arrhythmias? Any ischemic changes?
CXR	Cardiomegaly or any other signs of heart disease? Pneumonia?

MI, myocardial infarction; UTI, urinary tract infection; HIV, human immunodeficiency virus; CNS, central nervous system; ECG, electroencephalogram; CXR, chest x-ray study.

obtained to visualize the brainstem, the cerebellum, and the eighth cranial nerve in much better detail.

Assessment

As mentioned in the introduction, the first major determination in a patient presenting with "dizziness" is to precisely characterize the symptoms as vertigo or light-headedness.

Vertigo

Vertigo can be caused by peripheral lesions (i.e., inner ear or eighth cranial nerve) or central lesions (brainstem and cerebellum). Clues from the

TABLE 8-3
Imaging Tests to Work up Dizziness

Modality	Results
MRI/MRA with contrast	Should include stroke sequences (DWI, ADC maps) and perfusion where available. In cases in which a posterior circulation stroke is suspected, it is absolutely necessary.
CT scan	Useful in identifying brainstem hemorrhages and some vascular malformations, and large mass lesions impinging on cranial nerve VIII and the brainstem. CT scan with contrast may reveal a brain abscess and other mass lesions such as toxoplasmosis and lymphoma.
CT angiogram	If a posterior circulation vascular event is suspected, a CT angiogram may be useful in determining the patency of the posterior circulation.

DWI, diffusion-weighted imaging; ADC, apparent diffusion coefficent; CT, computed tomography.

history, physical exam, and ancillary testing help you localize the lesion. Once you have localized the lesion to either a peripheral or a central cause, the differential diagnosis can be considered. Table 8-4 lists the most common causes of vertigo by localization. Explanations of some of these causes follow.

Peripheral Causes of Vertigo. The most common peripheral causes of vertigo are the following:

- Benign paroxysmal positional vertigo (BPPV). BPPV is a common cause of peripheral vertigo, accounting for about 20% of all patients with dizziness. It is caused by calcium carbonate crystals (otoconia) that are dislodged and collect within the canals, in turn causing inappropriate cupula movement with changes in static head posture. BPPV presents with vertigo, imbalance, and nausea and vomiting that last up to a minute, induced by abrupt changes of the position of the head relative to gravity. Episodes are characterized by the following:
  - Brevity (i.e., last just seconds)
  - Latency to the vertigo and nystagmus (usually seconds)

TABLE 8-4
Common Causes of Vertigo by Localization

Central	Peripheral
Stroke	Benign paroxysmal positional vertigo (BPPV)
Demyelinating disease such as multiple sclerosis	Vestibular or acoustic neuritis
Abscess	Ménière's disease
Migraine	Acoustic neuroma
Vitamin B1 deficiency	Posttraumatic

- Fatigability with repetitive positioning
- Nystagmus that is mixed vertical/torsional beating upwards in the orbit with torsion beating toward the dependent ear
- The Dix-Hallpike maneuver is used to induce nystagmus (Fig. 8-1). Do not attempt this maneuver unless supervised by another physician because of the potential danger of neck injury by turning the patient's head.
- Vestibular or acoustic neuritis. Vestibular neuronitis, also called acoustic neuronitis, is characterized by acute episodes of vertigo that are spontaneous, even with the head still, but that are usually worsened by head movement. It may last hours to days, and at least initially presents with nausea and vomiting. It may also recur. Its cause is thought to be infectious/inflammatory. Ramsay Hunt syndrome is a form of otic herpes zoster infection that affects the cranial nerves VII and VIII. It generally presents with ear pain followed by a vesicular eruption within the external auditory canal.
- Ménière's disease. Ménière's disease is characterized by episodes of severe vertigo that usually last a day or two and that are usually preceded by pain, pressure, or fullness in the ear, as well as by fluctuating hearing loss and tinnitus. The cause is thought be an increase in endolymph pressure.
- Tumor or masses. Acoustic schwannomas or other tumors affecting the eighth cranial nerve are usually found in the cerebello-pontine angle.
- Posttraumatic vertigo. This may be seen up to several days after head trauma and is thought to be a form of peripheral vertigo, similar to a BPPV-like syndrome. It may resolve on its own after a week, but if vertigo persists, a complete workup with imaging should be considered. Perilymphatic fistula as a sequela from trauma is rare and is usually associated with hearing loss.

Central Causes of Vertigo. The most common central causes of vertigo are the following:

- Stroke. Acute vertigo often presents in the context of a lateral medullary or brainstem cerebrovascular event associated with ipsilateral ataxia, Horner's syndrome, skew deviation of the eyes with a head-tilt oscillopsia, ipsilateral facial sensation loss, and a contralateral loss of sensation of the body. It is associated with loss of flow from the posterior inferior cerebellar artery or basilar artery.
- Cerebellar infarction or hemorrhage. A cerebellar infarction or hemorrhage may present with isolated vertigo (distal posterior inferior cerebellar artery [PICA] syndrome, also known as Wallenberg's syndrome).
- Multiple sclerosis. Demyelinating lesions in the brainstem can cause eye findings and vertigo. When it affects the vestibular nucleus, it leads to vertigo. Although plaques may form anywhere in the brainstem, a typical lesion involving the medial longitudinal fasciculus causes loss of lateral conjugate gaze. As lateral gaze begins, the affected adducting eye fails to follow the abducting one, causing diplopia. On extreme gaze, nystagmus of the abducting eye will appear. Thus these lesions will manifest as vertigo plus the previously mentioned eye findings.
- Vertiginous migraine. Vertigo associated with migraine headache in a stereotypical, repetitive pattern is common in migraineurs and in families with a history of migraines.

CLINICAL PEARL

Occasionally, vertiginous migraine may present with vertigo without headache, but such a diagnosis should be reserved as a diagnosis of exclusion.

Time Course of Symptoms of Vertigo. The time course of symptoms can also provide some clues to the cause (Table 8-5).

TABLE 8-5

The Cause of Vertigo Based on the Time Course of Symptoms

Acute	Episodic
Vestibular or acoustic neuritis	BPPV
Stroke	Recurrent TIA
	Migraine
	Ménière's Disease
	Acoustic neuroma

Light-headedness

Common causes of light-headedness are generally limited to three problems:

- Neurologic causes. Neurologic causes present as hypoperfusion to the brainstem or cerebral cortex. Workup and treatment should be focused on vascular risk factors.
- Cardiogenic causes or orthostatic hypotension. These causes result in a feeling of light-headedness or tunnel vision and are usually induced by standing up suddenly. It generally lasts a few seconds and may eventually lead to a full syncopal episode with loss of consciousness.
- Psychiatric causes. Anxiety and depression, usually chronic, may result in odd symptoms, such as a feeling of floating or weightlessness.

Treatment

The treatment of dizziness focuses on treating the underlying causes:

- Stroke. Basilar artery occlusion and cerebellar hemorrhage or infarction require emergent care. If within the timeframe of 3 hours from the onset of attack or the time the patient was last seen as normal, *intravenous* rt-TPA should be considered. *Intra-arterial* TPA can be administered within a 6-hour timeframe. If outside the timeframes, other recanalization strategies such as mechanical methods should be considered.
- Vertiginous migraine. Prophylactic therapy with calcium channel blockers has been proven to be effective.
- Orthostatic hypotension. The mainline treatment is rehydration, preferably by administering fluids, but in cases of vertigo with nausea, usually intravenous hydration is necessary.
- Vestibular neuritis. The mechanism of injury has been proposed to involve either viral infection with a member of the herpes family or inflammation. Starting a prednisone taper within 3 days of the start of symptoms has been shown to provide some benefit; however, antivirals such as acyclovir have not been proven to be effective. It is important to rule out a bacterial infection. If one is suspected, then appropriate antibiotics need to be started. In addition, the patient may need to be admitted for rehydration and may need to be administered an adequate antiemetic regimen. Vestibular suppression medications should be used judiciously because they can cause sedation and can alter the neurologic exam. The length of use is debatable, but most specialists would not recommend more than 5 days, at which point if symptoms do not improve, the patient may need to be re-evaluated.
- BPPV. Epley positioning maneuver may be attempted along with vestibular suppression medication.
- Mass effect on the brainstem. If an abscess is suspected, then antibiotics need to be started (be watchful for toxoplasmosis in patients who are HIV positive). If a neoplasm is present with edema, then steroids are an option.

- Ménière's disease. In the acute setting, antihistamines, sedatives (benzodiazepines), and anticholinergics (such as a Scopoderm patch) can be used for symptomatic control. Long-term intratympanic injections with gentamicin or surgical intervention may be necessary to provide relief.
- Posttraumatic vertigo. In the acute setting, antihistamines and anticholinergics may be used.

EXTENDED INHOSPITAL MANAGEMENT

Inhospital management for patients with dizziness initially focuses on ruling out life-threatening conditions. Laboratory testing and imaging should be completed within 24 to 48 hours, and the differential diagnosis can be narrowed to a few likely conditions. There are a few conditions in which extended inpatient treatment may be necessary. These include the following:

- Intracranial hemorrhage
- Brainstem stroke or thrombosis
- Uncharacterized inflammatory disorder

For treatment of vertigo owing to peripheral causes, a short inpatient hospitalization serves to stabilize the patient and rehydrate him or her as necessary. Vestibular therapy is helpful in teaching patients to deal with chronic vertigo. Therapy can be started on an inpatient basis (if available) and continued on an outpatient basis.

DISPOSITION

Discharge Goals

The goal of discharging a patient with dizziness is to discover the cause, stabilize the condition, and begin treatment. A workup for life-threatening causes of dizziness should be ruled out or managed by day of discharge. Symptomatic treatment with antiemetics may be necessary to allow the patient to return to work.

Outpatient Care

Many of the causes of peripheral vertigo are managed in the outpatient setting by the primary care physician along with a general neurologist. Chronic or relapsing BBPV, chronic labyrinthitis, and intractable Ménière's disease may require consultation with an otorhinolaryngologist or specialized vestibular neurologist. Rarely, migraines that are difficult to control may require the consultation of a neurologist who specializes in headaches.

For patients with neurologic causes of light-headedness caused by vasculopathy, such as atherosclerosis of the posterior circulation, regular outpatient visits with a neurologist or a primary care physician are essential to successfully modifying vascular risk factors such as hypertension, diabetes, and hypercholesterolemia. Orthostatic hypotension can be well managed by a primary care physician, but there are autonomic neurologic specialists who can provide insights into complicated cases.

WHAT YOU NEED TO REMEMBER

- Dizziness can be characterized as either vertigo or light-headedness. Vertigo is the inappropriate sensation of movement, such as spinning, whereas light-headedness is a feeling of faintness.
- Vertigo can be localized to the circuit encompassing the inner ear, the eighth cranial nerve, the brainstem, and the deep cerebellar nuclei. Light-headedness can localize to the posterior circulation but can also be caused by general systemic abnormalities such as medication toxicity.
- Patients presenting with acute vertigo or light-headedness should be ruled out for life-threatening conditions, including basilar thrombosis and brainstem stroke.
- The history and physical exam are key to localizing a neurologic lesion. Imaging and labs can be helpful for diagnosing certain conditions.
- Treatments for vertigo and light-headedness depend on the specific cause. Once the patient is stabilized and discharged home, most causes of dizziness (vertigo and light-headedness) can be managed on an outpatient basis.

SUGGESTED READINGS

Furman JM, Cass SP. *Vestibular Disorders: A Case Study Approach.* 2nd Ed. New York: Oxford University Press, USA, 2002.

Lustig L, Niparko J, Minor LB, et al. *Clinical Neurotology: Diagnosing and Managing Disorders of Hearing, Balance and the Facial Nerve.* 1st Ed. London, UK: Informa Healthcare, 2002.

Visual Changes

THE PATIENT ENCOUNTER

An 80-year-old man presents with a sudden loss of vision in the right eye. He says he was watching TV when he suddenly noticed that he could not see anything out of his right eye. He has no other complaints.

OVERVIEW

Definition and Pathophysiology

Most complaints about visual changes can be organized into three categories: (i) loss of vision (complete or incomplete), (ii) problems with eye movements (disorders of ocular motility), and (iii) visual hallucinations or other positive visual phenomena. To diagnose the cause of visual impairment, it is important not only to take a comprehensive history and perform a good neurologic exam, but also to understand anatomy of the eye, the visual pathway in the brain, pupillary innervation, and the anatomy of visual tracts in the brainstem. Loss of vision can originate from a lesion in the orbit or brain. Pupillary dysfunction can come from lesions in the orbit, brain, brainstem, or the extracranial sympathetic system. Localization of changes in vision is based on the clinical history and the combination of findings of the neurologic exam.

Once the anatomic location of the lesion is identified, the cause can be investigated. Etiology varies widely depending on the location of the lesion, but visual changes can be a result of vascular disease, infection, malignancy, demyelination, trauma, toxic exposure, degenerative disease, inflammatory disease, metabolic derangement, or systemic disease.

In this chapter, we will discuss the evaluation of patients who present with complaints of visual loss or problems with ocular motility. Positive visual phenomena can result from orbital pathology (retinal detachment), parenchymal pathology (migraines, occipital lobe strokes, and occipital lobe seizures), or drug effect (alcohol withdrawal). This particular complaint will be touched on in other chapters; it is usually accompanied by other localizing signs and symptoms.

Epidemiology

People of any age can have visual disturbances. However, certain visual complaints are more common among certain age groups. It is important that the age, sex, and race of the patient will help narrow, or at least prioritize, the differential diagnosis for his or her visual problem. We might suspect vascular disease as the most likely cause for monocular vision loss in an 80-year-old man, whereas demyelinating disease would be most likely in a 25-year-old woman with the same complaint.

ACUTE MANAGEMENT AND WORKUP

A few situations require emergent workup and management that must begin in the emergency department but can be completed in an inpatient setting.

The First 15 Minutes

Vision loss is a symptom that prompts immediate concern to the patient, and often the patient presents very early in the course of illness. The first 15 minutes of the evaluation should focus on potentially reversing the disease course and restoring the patient's vision.

Initial Assessment

The first question that one should ask in the initial evaluation of the patient is *Does this patient potentially need acute intervention to help with diagnosis or management?* When dealing with vision, there are a few emergent situations. For example, symptoms that could be attributable to ischemic or hemorrhagic stroke should be evaluated immediately because vision loss caused by an infarct of the optic nerve or brain can potentially be reversible. Diplopia or vision loss owing to an infarct in the brainstem could be reversible, but more important, could be the first clue that the patient is at risk to have a much larger brainstem stroke in the immediate future. If pseudotumor is the suspected cause for visual loss, permanent visual loss can potentially be prevented by cerebrospinal fluid (CSF) drainage. If myasthenia gravis is suspected, the patient should be evaluated for pulmonary function, as respiratory failure in patients with myasthenia can be sudden.

The following visual complaints necessitate emergent evaluation:

- *Hemianopia or quadrantanopsia owing to a hemorrhagic or ischemic stroke.* Strokes, whether hemorrhagic or ischemic, should be monitored carefully in an inpatient setting. Depending on the nature and location of the stroke, certain blood pressure parameters should be set immediately. In addition, if the stroke is ischemic and has happened within the last 3 hours, *intravenous* tPA (tissue plasminogen activator) can be considered to lyse the clot. If it has happened within the last 6 hours, *intra-arterial* tPA directly into the thrombosed artery is a treatment option if available at the hospital.
- *Unilateral visual loss owing to acute ischemic optic neuropathy.* If caused by occlusion of the central retinal artery, intra-arterial tPA might restore vision if administered within a reasonable period of time (see previous paragraph).
- *Unilateral or bilateral blurry vision owing to pseudotumor cerebri.* Because visual loss can be permanent, urgent CSF drainage is often indicated in these situations.

- *Acute-onset double vision or nystagmus that could be localizable to the brainstem.* If acute onset symptoms *could* be owing to an ischemic stroke in the midbrain or pons, patients should have emergent evaluations of the posterior cerebral circulation via CT (CT angiogram), MR (MR angiogram), or conventional angiogram, depending on the availability at your hospital. Brainstem strokes can be tricky to diagnose; symptoms can wax and wane and can be nonspecific, and strokes can ultimately be devastating or potentially fatal. Intra-arterial tPA can be used in cases of basilar artery occlusion to help restore blood flow.
- *Visual symptoms possibly related to myasthenia gravis.* Patients should have pulmonary function tests performed immediately to determine whether or not this flare of their disease may lead to acute neuromuscular respiratory failure and a need for intubation.

Admission Criteria and Level of Care Criteria

The second question you should ask is *Does this symptom necessitate hospital admission, or can workup and treatment be done on an outpatient basis?* In general, when confronted with a visual complaint, admission is warranted. Exceptions are as follows:

- Symptoms that have been going on for weeks to months that have not worsened recently. For example, someone with double vision owing to a suspected oculomotor nerve palsy whose symptoms began 1 month ago and have not changed is not at high risk for worsening of the symptoms in the immediate future. This patient can be evaluated in the outpatient neurology or ophthalmology clinic.
- Symptoms with a known cause based on the patient's prior history that can be treated on an outpatient basis. For example, patients with known demyelinating disease who present with optic neuritis can be treated with IV steroids at home.

The First 24 Hours

The remainder of visual complaints thought to need urgent workup should be evaluated via laboratory workup, imaging, and possibly lumbar puncture in a nonemergent inpatient setting.

History

Obtaining a comprehensive history is the most important step in diagnosing the cause for a change in vision. When exploring visual loss, the following questions should be addressed:

- For all visual complaints:
  - Was the onset acute, subacute, or chronic?
  - Is it monocular or binocular?
  - Are symptoms constant or do they wax and wane?

- Is there associated eye pain?
- Is there an associated headache?
- For complaints of visual loss:
  - Is it complete loss or partial loss, and if partial, where is the deficit?
- For complaints of double vision:
  - Is double vision vertical, horizontal, or otherwise?

The remainder of the history should be taken with special attention to the following:

- Review of systems. Are there associated fever, chills, or other signs/symptoms of infection? Has there been weight loss or fatigue, which is suggestive of a systemic process?
- Past medical history. Is there a history of other ocular or visual problems? Does the patient have vascular disease or risk factors for vascular disease? Is there a history of autoimmune or inflammatory diseases? Does the patient have a history of headaches? Is there a history of malignancies? Has there been recent trauma?
- Medications. Have there been recent changes in the patient's medication regimen?
- Family history. Are there other family members who have had similar complaints in the past?
- Social history. Has the patient had any possible exposure to toxins?

Physical Examination

Physical examination should focus on visual acuity, visual field testing, pupillary responses, extraocular movements, funduscopic examination, and careful examination of the remaining cranial nerves.

- *Visual acuity.* Visual acuity can be tested with a Snellen or Rosenbaum eye chart. One eye should be tested at a time, and testing should be performed with glasses on. If vision is so poor that neither eye chart is useful, the ability of the patient to count fingers (CF), detect hand movement (HM), or perceive light should be recorded. If an eye is totally blind, NLP (no light perception) should be noted. If visual acuity is reasonably good bilaterally and there is a history that suggests an optic nerve lesion, red desaturation should be tested. If a patient looks at the same red object with one eye and then the other, and the shade of red appears dull when looking with the affected eye, it is suggestive of optic neuropathy in that eye.
- *Visual fields.* Visual field testing should also be performed on each eye separately. With visual field testing, the examiner should note a pattern of deficit and whether it is monocular or binocular. A central scotoma or complete loss of vision in one eye suggests an optic nerve lesion. A partial optic nerve lesion can cause a monocular hemianopia. Optic chiasm lesions classically cause bitemporal hemianopia. Lesions in the optic tract

cause homonymous hemianopias, whereas lesions of the optic radiations cause homonymous hemianopias (larger lesions) or quadrantanopsias (smaller lesions). A posterior cerebral artery infarction causes a homonymous hemianopia with macular sparing in that patients retain central vision but lose all peripheral vision.

• Pupillary reaction to light should be tested with a bright light.

> ### CLINICAL PEARL
>
> *Common pen lights are often too dull to elicit a maximal pupillary response. Consider investing in a halogen pen light.*

A unilateral nonreactive pupil can result from disease of the iris (glaucoma) or optic nerve (ischemia, infarction, demyelination). Light–near dissociation is an absence of pupillary reaction to light but a brisk constriction to accommodation (focusing on a near object); it is classically associated with neurosyphilis, but is also caused by diabetes, optic nerve disease, or tumors that compress the midbrain tectum. Argyll Robertson pupils are small, irregularly shaped, and poorly reactive to light. Neurosyphilis or other diseases that affect the Edinger-Westphal nucleus can be the cause. If a miotic pupil (a small, unreactive pupil) is associated with ptosis and possibly anhidrosis, Horner's syndrome is the likely culprit. Horner's syndrome can be from a lesion in the hypothalamus or brainstem, preganglionic neuron in the stellate ganglion in the chest, or postganglionic neuron in the cavernous sinus. Rapid afferent pupillary defect (RAPD) is a condition in which an optic nerve is unable to carry light information back to the Edinger-Westphal nucleus. On exam, an RAPD is manifested as bilaterally reactive pupils when light is shined in the good eye and bilateral *un*reactive pupils when light is shined in the bad eye. RAPD is commonly seen in patients with acute or chronic optic neuritis.

• *Extraocular movements.* When extraocular movements are observed, particular attention should be paid to the extremes of gaze, and you should ask about diplopia throughout this part of the exam. As part of the evaluation of extraocular movements, saccades (horizontal and vertical) should be tested. Limitations of gaze may help identify a specific extraocular nerve palsy. Nystagmus can be suggestive of peripheral or central vestibular dysfunction or the toxic effects of drugs such as phenytoin (see Chapter 8, Dizziness). Vertical misalignment of the eyes usually suggests a brainstem lesion.

• *Funduscopic exam.* Funduscopic examination should also be performed on every patient with visual complaints. You should note disc pallor (suggestive of prior optic nerve injury), the blurring of disc margins (suggestive of papilledema), the presence or absence of venous pulsations (a lack of which can indicate increased intracranial pressure), and macular pathology (as one might expect in macular degeneration).

• *Cranial nerves.* Examination of the remainder of the nervous system, with special attention paid to cranial nerves, can help localize a neurologic lesion, especially if more than one cranial nerve is involved. One of the classic brainstem stroke syndromes, lateral medullary syndrome (Wallenberg syndrome) results from a posterior inferior cerebellar artery occlusion, which causes the following: (i) ipsilateral cerebellar ataxia, Horner's syndrome, and facial sensory deficit; (ii) contralateral impaired pain and temperature sensation; and (iii) nystagmus, vertigo, nausea, vomiting, dysphagia, dysarthria, and hiccups.

Between the history and the physical exam, a visual lesion can usually be localized or localization can be narrowed down to a few different anatomic regions. Once a location is suspected, the causes can be explored. For potential causes of visual abnormalities resulting from specifically localized lesions, please refer to Tables 9-2 and 9-3 in the Assessment section of this chapter.

Labs and Tests to Consider

Laboratory workup should be initiated in the emergency room or clinic setting, but results are not always crucial in deciding a patient's disposition.

Key Diagnostic Labs and Tests

For the significance of abnormal lab results, refer to Table 9-1. Lumbar puncture (LP) should be urgently performed (after head imaging is done to ensure safety of the LP) if a patient might potentially have pseudotumor cerebri or a central nervous system (CNS) infection. If demyelinating or degenerative disease is suspected, an LP should be performed, but it does not need to be done urgently.

Imaging and Ancillary Testing

Although imaging is often helpful with localization and in defining the cause in neurologic illnesses, it is rarely diagnostic in the setting of visual complaints. All patients who present with acute-onset visual symptoms should have a CT scan of the head performed in the emergency department. This is critical in identifying bleeds (subarachnoid blood that causes a cranial nerve palsy or intraparenchymal blood that causes a visual field cut) and might be helpful in identifying an intracranial malignancy (a tumor encroaching on optic pathway). Rarely, however, is a CT diagnostic in non-hemorrhagic causes of visual complaints. In some cases, MRI of the orbits, brain, and brainstem with and without contrast can be useful to help identify common causes of visual abnormalities, including parenchymal ischemic stroke, malignancy, loci of an infection, or evidence of other brain pathology. If a vascular cause for visual loss is suggested by history and examination, a

TABLE 9-1

Key Laboratory Tests and Rationales for Testing

Test	Significance
Serum Tests	
Elevated WBC count	Infection, vascular disease, malignancy
Decreased WBC count	Immunosuppressed state suggesting susceptibility to infections, malignancy
Increased glucose	History of diabetes
Elevated INR or aPTT ratio	Predisposition to bleeding, possible use of Coumadin
Elevated liver function tests and/or abnormal coagulation rates	Underlying liver disease suggestive of alcohol use, exposure to hepatotoxic drugs
Elevated ANA	Inflammatory or autoimmune disease
Elevated ESR or CRP	Infection, autoimmune disease, inflammatory disease (temporal arteritis), malignancy
Spinal Fluid Tests	
Elevated opening pressure	Pseudotumor cerebri or CNS infection
Elevated WBC count	Infection, demyelination, or inflammatory disease
Low glucose	Bacterial or fungal infection
Elevated protein	Infection, demyelination, inflammatory disease, or tumor
Elevated IgG or IgG index	Demyelination
Presence of oligoclonal bands	Demyelination

WBC, white blood count; INR, international normalized ratio; aPTT, activated partial thromboplastin time; ANA, antinuclear antibody; ESR, erythrocyte sedimentation rate; CRP, C-reactive protein; CNS, central nervous system; IgG, immunoglobulin G.

CT angiogram, an MR angiogram, or a conventional angiogram can help diagnose aneurysms, vascular malformations, and dissections.

Assessment

The key to determining the cause of the visual complaint is localization of the lesion. The history, physical exam, and ancillary testing provide the clues. Table 9-2 lists the most common causes of visual loss based on localization of

TABLE 9-2
Differential Diagnoses of Visual Loss

Localization	Cause
Retina	Retinal detachment Infection (CMV, toxoplasmosis) Toxicity (ethambutol) Degenerative (macular degeneration)
Optic disc	Acute ischemic optic neuropathy Optic neuritis Glaucoma Pseudotumor cerebri Sarcoidosis Tumor
Optic nerve	Demyelination (multiple sclerosis, neuromyelitis optica) Thyroid disease Trauma Tumor
Chiasm	Aneurysm (internal carotid artery [ICA]) Demyelination (multiple sclerosis) Vascular disease Toxicity Trauma Tumor
Retrochiasmal	Vascular disease (stroke) or reversible posterior leukoencephalopathy (RPLE) Demyelination (multiple sclerosis) Degenerative disease Tumor

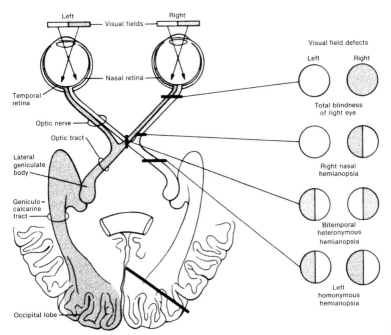

FIGURE 9-1: Lesions in the optic pathways. The anatomy of the optic nerves (prechiasmal) and tracts (postchiasmal) explains the visual field deficit. A lesion in the optic nerve can affect all vision from only the ipsilateral eye, but a partial optic nerve lesion can present with a visual field loss. A lesion in the center of the optic chiasm causes bitemporal hemianopia because only the tracts of the crossing medial nerves are affected. An optic tract lesion causes homonymous hemianopia because it contains the medial tracts from the contralateral eye (carrying visual information from the temporal field of the contralateral eye) plus the lateral tracts from the ipsilateral eye (carrying visual information from the medial field of the ipsilateral eye). Lesions affecting the entire occipital lobe also present with homonymous hemianopias. From Harwood-Nuss A, et al. *The Clinical Practice of Emergency Medicine,* 3rd Ed. Philadelphia: Lippincott Williams & Wilkins, 2001.

the lesion from the retina to the occipital cortex in the back of the brain (retrochiasmal). In thinking about the localization of lesions causing visual field deficits, it is helpful to use the diagram in Figure 9-1 to understand the anatomy. Table 9-3 lists the most common causes of diplopia.

Treatment

In the field of medicine, neurologists and ophthalmologist have generally divided their territory at the start of the optic nerve. Anything having to the do with the eye itself, including the retina, is the responsibility of the ophthalmologist. All other disorders of vision that are localized anywhere

TABLE 9-3
Differential Diagnoses of Diplopia

Localization	Cause
Extraocular muscle	Thyroid disease Degenerative disease (muscular dystrophy)
Neuromuscular junction	Myasthenia gravis Paraneoplastic disease (Lambert-Eaton syndrome)
Oculomotor nerves	Vascular disease (ischemia, diabetes, vasculitis) Aneurysm Trauma Tumor Infection (syphilis, Lyme) Demyelination (multiple sclerosis)
Central nuclei	Demyelination (multiple sclerosis) Vascular disease Sarcoidosis Tumor
Central connections	Demyelination Vascular disease Sarcoidosis Tumor

behind the eye, including the optic nerves, the optic chiasm, optic tracts, the brainstem, and the brain, are the responsibility of the neurologist. Shared territory includes disorders involving the orbit, the extraocular muscles, and cranial nerves III, IV, and VI. For this chapter, we will focus on treatments of neurologic diseases of vision.

Table 9-4 lists the diseases from Tables 9-2 and 9-3 and divides them into treatment categories.

EXTENDED INHOSPITAL MANAGEMENT

Inhospital management should focus on the diagnosis and the initiation of treatment. Diagnostic tests not emergently needed (i.e., MRI of the brain,

TABLE 9-4
Treatment of Visual Loss and Diplopia

Category of Disease	Diseases	Treatment
Vascular	Acute ischemic optic neuropathy, vasculitis, diabetes; aneurysm; RPLE	In the acute setting, consider thrombolysis; long-term modification of vascular risk factors; aneurysms need neurosurgical evaluation for clipping vs. coiling; RPLE demands aggressive blood pressure control
Infectious	Syphilis, Lyme, toxoplasmosis, CMV	Antimicrobial therapy with ophthalmologic consultation
Trauma	Trauma	Acutely stabilize and control bleeding
Inflammatory	Optic neuritis, Sarcoidosis, demyelinating disease	Acutely treat with steroids; long-term immunosuppression may be necessary
Metabolic	Thyroid disease; drug toxicity (ethambutol)	Thyroid disease should be evaluated and treated by endocrinologist; in suspected drug toxicity, drug should be discontinued immediately
Neoplastic	Tumor, paraneoplastic	For tumor, obtain neurosurgical consult (may or may not require surgery); for paraneoplastic disorder, plasma exchange may be best therapy after removal of primary tumor

RPLE, reversible posterior leukoencephalopathy; CMV, cytomegalovirus.

lumbar puncture) can be done after the patient is admitted. Some patients do not receive diagnoses right away, but this should not prolong their hospital stay. The goal of hospitalization is to rule out diagnoses that need prompt attention. For example, if a patient comes in with visual loss thought to be caused by optic neuritis but neither MRI nor LP hints at a specific demyelinating disease, he or she can go home once treatment with IV steroids has been initiated (or completed). A diagnosis may become obvious with additional testing on an outpatient basis or with the passage of time.

DISPOSITION

Discharge Goals

At the end of a hospital stay, all life-threatening and potentially reversible causes of visual loss should be addressed, and patients should be otherwise stable. Workup and/or treatment can be continued once the patient goes home if he or she does not need to be monitored in a hospital setting.

Outpatient Care

Follow-up depends on the cause of the visual symptoms. Appropriate follow-up may be arranged with any of the following types of specialties, either individually or in any combination: ophthalmology, neurology, neurosurgery, oncology, infectious disease, rheumatology, and endocrinology.

WHAT YOU NEED TO REMEMBER

- Visual changes are grouped into three categories: loss of vision, double vision, and hallucinations (gain of vision). Loss of vision can be caused by a lesion anywhere between the eye and the visual cortex. Double vision is usually an eye motility issue. Hallucinations or bright flashes always localize to the retina or cortex.
- Ophthalmologists handle everything within the eye; neurologists handle everything from the optic nerve to the brain.
- Localization of the lesion is the first and most important step in diagnosing a visual problem. Each segment of the visual pathway is susceptible to common disorders.
- Acute vision loss can be potentially reversible if diagnosed and treated quickly.

SUGGESTED READINGS

Aminoff MJ, Greenberg DA, Simon RP. *Clinical Neurology*. 6th Ed. New York: Lange Medical Books/McGraw-Hill, 2005.

Brazis PW, Masdeau JC, Biller J. *Localization in Clinical Neurology*. 6th Ed. Philadelphia: Lippincott Williams & Wilkins, 2006.

Patten JP. *Neurological Differential Diagnosis*. 2nd Ed. New York: Springer, 1998.

Headache and Facial Pain

THE PATIENT ENCOUNTER

A 45-year-old woman comes to the emergency room after abrupt onset of pounding pain over her left temple that started 30 minutes ago. She feels generally bad, diffusely achy, and cognitively cloudy. She also reports light and sound sensitivity and mild nausea, but no vomiting. She has a neck ache, but she has not had a fever.

OVERVIEW

Definition and Pathophysiology

Pain in the head or face can be attributed to any of the structures in the head except the brain itself. The sensation of pain requires pain-sensitive nerve endings, which are present in the blood vessels, meninges, muscle, bone, and skin of the head and face but are not present within the brain parenchyma. Therefore, headache pain is produced by derangement of the blood vessels, meninges, muscle, bone, and skin of the head.

The International Headache Society broadly divides headaches into two etiologic categories: primary and secondary. Primary headache syndromes, which include migraine, tension headache, and cluster headache, are common, can seriously detract from the quality of life, and are a major cause of impaired productivity worldwide, but are not immediately life-threatening. Most prominent among the primary headache syndromes, migraine is thought to develop through a neurovascular mechanism. In this process, a wave of excitation spreads across the cortex, usually beginning in the occipital region. This wave leads to consequent vasomotor spasms, which are painful. Although migraine pain is owing to pain from vascular spasm, PET (positron emission tomography) studies have revealed that the wave of excitation crosses cerebrovascular territories, suggesting that a primary pathology may be within the cortex itself. Patients with primary headache syndromes tend, on careful questioning, to have had similar headaches before and can usually describe several headache triggers.

In contrast, the secondary headache syndromes are most important to identify emergently because when they present acutely or subacutely, they can be life threatening. Secondary headache syndromes are caused by pathologic processes as diverse as subarachnoid, subdural, or epidural hemorrhages; brain tumors; meningitis; and temporal arteritis. Again, the common thread is that pain is generated through derangement of pain-sensing structures within the blood vessels, meninges, muscle, bone, and skin of the head. A triggering event may or may not be identifiable. Keep in mind that patients with primary headache syndromes can have secondary headaches, too, and may have acquired a chronic primary headache syndrome from a secondary cause.

Red flags for dangerous headaches are sudden onset, change in headache pattern, new-onset headaches in someone with no history of headaches (especially in a patient older than 50 years of age), the presence of systemic illness, malaise, nausea, vomiting (especially in the morning), stiff neck, fever, or the presence of medical illness with frequent neurologic complications, such as cancer or HIV.

Epidemiology

Among all complaints, headaches are the ninth most common chief complaint in the primary care setting. Headaches are common among all ages, but *new-onset* headaches in anyone older than 50 years of age is unusual and should prompt a thorough workup.

ACUTE MANAGEMENT AND WORKUP

Your four-step approach to a patient with headache is as follows:

1. Use the first 15 minutes to ensure that your patient is stable.
2. When stable, take time to obtain a complete history, perform a thorough physical examination, send lab tests, and obtain a noncontrast (dry) head CT.
3. Formulate an assessment that involves localizing the lesion and developing a differential diagnosis.
4. Discuss the case with neurology or neurosurgery and establish a treatment plan.

The First 15 Minutes

The goal of the first 15 minutes in evaluating a patient with chief complaint of headache is to rule out a life-threatening condition that could rapidly worsen. Always consider life-threatening conditions in any patient with headache, even if he or she has a history of benign headaches. For example, in the patient encounter above, the 45-year-old woman may have a history of tension headaches, but this presentation should not be dismissed as another tension headache; rather, this woman needs a rapid evaluation and workup for infectious and vascular causes of headache that are life-threatening.

Initial Assessment

When you first see a patient with a headache, you first want to assess airway, breathing, and circulation, as in all potentially emergent situations. In the secondary assessment, pay closer attention to the vital signs, looking for fever, hypertension, bradycardia, tachycardia, or abnormalities in the respiratory rate or pattern. With these initial assessments, you will establish if the patient is hemodynamically stable and determine if the patient is in imminent danger. Ask the question: *Is this patient going to die or suffer severe disability in the next few minutes if you do not intervene?*

Look for the following emergent signs that require immediate attention:

1. Dilated, asymmetrical, unreactive, or pinpoint pupils (signs of serious cranial nerve or brainstem dysfunction)
2. Neck stiffness (sign of meningeal irritation from subarachnoid hemorrhage or infection)
3. Fever ($\geq$38°C or 100.4°F) (sign of infection)
4. High blood pressure, low heart rate, irregular respirations (signs of high intracranial pressure—Cushing's triad)
5. Ongoing seizure activity (status epilepticus)
6. Complaints of rapidly progressive blindness (sign of temporal arteritis, high intracranial pressure, or occipital lobe dysfunction)

Admission Criteria and Level of Care Criteria

Patients with acute headache should be admitted; patients with chronic headaches can be managed on an outpatient basis but should be admitted if their headache pattern is new or suspicious. "Worst headache ever," a new headache in a patient older than 50 years of age, a new headache pattern, and morning headaches are concerning symptoms. Migraines are almost always associated with photophobia/phonophobia, and nausea and vomiting. In the absence of these symptoms, migraine should not be at the top of your list of differential diagnosis. Migraines that present with focal neurologic symptoms (formerly known as *complicated migraines*) should be evaluated for stroke or other mass lesion.

The First 24 Hours

In the first 24 hours of admission, the goal is to obtain all testing needed to help make the diagnosis and begin treatment.

History

If the patient is unstable, obtain a focused history from family (only 1 and 2 in the list that follows), and proceed to physical exam. If the patient is stable but not conversant, obtain a history from a family member or friend. If the patient is stable, awake, and conversant, obtain a full history directly from the patient.

- *Headache pattern and character*. Determine the headache pattern and character by asking the patient the following questions:
  1. Is this the worst headache of the patient's life (think: subarachnoid hemorrhage)?
  2. Did the pain come on suddenly over seconds (think: hemorrhage), or gradually over minutes, hours, days, or weeks (think: tumor)?
  3. Is the headache present today only (secondary headache syndromes), every day (chronic daily headache), several days per month (migraine), or a certain part of every day (medication-related headache)?
  4. What parts of the head are involved?
  5. Is the pain constant, intermittent, throbbing, dull, sharp, or lancinating? Does the pain radiate anywhere else (carotid dissection pain often radiates anterior to the ear into the temple, and vertebral dissection pain radiates posterior to the ear over the occiput)? Is it position dependent (worse with lying down indicates high intracranial pressure; worse with standing up indicates low intracranial pressure)?
- *Associated symptoms*. Determine if the patient has had any of the following symptoms: nausea, vomiting, photophobia/phonophobia (think: migraine or subarachnoid hemorrhage), fever (think: meningitis), neck pain (think: meningitis or subarachnoid hemorrhage), malaise, arthralgias, visual changes, vision loss (think: temporal arteritis or pseudotumor cerebri), focal weakness or numbness (think: stroke, dissection, tumor, or hemorrhage), gait abnormalities (think: stroke or hydrocephalus), changes in sensation, or seizures (think: tumor or infection)
- *Headache history*. To establish a headache history, ask about the following:
  1. Is the patient a "headachy" person? Does he or she get migraines or regular headaches?
  2. How often does the patient have a headache and what are the usual associated symptoms?
  3. What headache triggers can the patient identify (alcohol, exercise, hunger, menstrual cycle, chocolate, certain smells)? Is this current presentation similar to his or her usual headaches?
- *Medication history*. Daily analgesic use can lead to chronic daily headaches owing to rebound headaches. Typical culprit analgesics include NSAIDs, over-the-counter migraine "cocktails," such as Tylenol Migraine and Excedrin (which also contains caffeine), narcotics, or any medicine that contains narcotics. Rebound headaches after treatment with narcotics are very common in migraine patients and should be avoided. A complete medication list should be obtained with special attention given to medication changes.
- *Social history*. Intravenous drug use can predispose to HIV infection and endocarditis, which can lead to stroke or hemorrhage. Cocaine use can cause vasospasm. Tobacco and alcohol history are also important for risk stratification. The patient's occupational history and history of recent trauma can also be important.

• *Family history*. Look for a history of headaches, aneurysms, and cancer specifically among other usual questions. Migraines run in families.

• *Neurologic review of systems.* Ask about a diminished level of consciousness at any point, vision changes, double vision, difficulty speaking, difficulty swallowing, facial asymmetry, focal weakness or numbness, gait disturbance, nausea, vomiting, vertigo, or seizures.

• *General review of systems.* Look for evidence of systemic illness. The date of the last menstrual period is important in migraineurs.

Physical Examination

After the primary and secondary assessments and history, examine the patient. Do both a focused medical examination and a careful neurologic examination.

During the medical exam, keep an eye on the patient's vital signs, and look for cachexia, rashes on the head or face, neck stiffness, pain to palpation of the skull or head and neck muscles, murmurs, or joint changes.

During the neurologic exam, first carefully examine the mental status. Is the patient awake? Does he or she arouse to voice, minor stimulation, or painful stimuli? Can he or she open the eyes and follow commands? Can he or she speak? Next, examine the cranial nerves. Do the pupils react? Are eye movements intact? Do a funduscopic exam looking for papilledema (a sign of elevated intracranial pressure). Is there ptosis? Nystagmus? Any facial asymmetry? Are gag and cough present? Move on to the motor exam: Can the patient move all four extremities and does he or she move them symmetrically? Does he or she withdraw, localize, or exhibit posturing to painful stimuli? If the patient is stable, check for abnormalities in gait and asymmetric reflexes.

Labs and Tests to Consider

Because headache is a nonspecific symptom that is caused by different diseases, labs and imaging studies are key to working up patients with headache. Depending on the suspected cause, lab and imaging tests should be prioritized. For example, in a patient with a suspected intracranial hemorrhage, a CT scan of the head should be obtained quickly. The next section presents lab and imaging tests for patients presenting with headache.

Key Diagnostic Labs and Tests

For patients with headache, a standard comprehensive metabolic panel and complete blood count with differential should be sent immediately. Additionally, toxicology and pregnancy screens are helpful. These will assess for toxic or metabolic causes of headaches. Furthermore, in older patients, an erythrocyte sedimentation rate (ESR) should be sent, in addition to a C-reactive protein (CRP). These studies are elevated in the setting of general inflammation, including inflammatory causes of headache, such as temporal arteritis and other vasculitides. An international normalized ratio (INR) and partial thromboplastin time ratio (PTTr) should also be sent in case the patient has a hemorrhage.

- If HIV risk factors are present, a rapid HIV test should be performed, if available. Determining HIV status is important for risk stratification in headache patients.
- If fever is present, blood and urine cultures should be drawn.
- If fever and/or neck stiffness are present, and the head CT is abnormal (for example, if subarachnoid blood or mass effect is observed), call neurology or neurosurgery immediately.
- If fever, neck stiffness, and/or peripheral leukocytosis are present, and the head CT is normal, perform lumbar puncture (LP). In headache patients, try to obtain an opening pressure. This measurement is accurate if the patient is lying on his or her side with legs extended. Normal values range from 8 to 20 cm H_2O.

Cerebrospinal fluid (CSF) studies should include cell count (white blood cells [WBCs], red blood cells [RBCs]), differential (polymorphonuclear [PMN] cells [neutrophils] and mononuclear cells [lymphocytes]), glucose, protein, Gram's stain, culture, herpes simplex virus polymer chain reaction (HSV PCR) and varicella-zoster virus PCR (VZV PCR). Do *not* delay antibiotic treatment if you suspect central nervous system (CNS) infection.

Imaging and Ancillary Testing

The next step is to obtain a noncontrast (dry) head CT. This test is easy to obtain quickly and is very sensitive for acute bleeds within the brain, such as intracerebral hemorrhage, subarachnoid hemorrhage, or subdural hemorrhage. The dry head CT may also demonstrate edema, hydrocephalus, or bone abnormalities that can suggest the cause of the headache.

If there is evidence of cerebrovascular dysfunction, such as stroke, carotid or vertebral dissection, or intracranial hemorrhage, a CT angiogram (CTA) of the head *and* neck can be helpful. CTAs can establish the patency of large intracranial and/or neck vessels. Arrange for a postcontrast image to look for blood-brain barrier breakdown caused by a tumor or inflammation.

MRI is the current gold standard for radiologic assessment of the central nervous system. However, because of the time required for adequate imaging and the cost of imaging, MRI is not the first line of imaging in the urgent setting. For optimal efficiency, MR studies should be ordered only after neurological or neurosurgical consultation. MRI should be performed with and without gadolinium (Gd^{3+}) contrast. In parts of the brain where there is breakdown of the blood-brain barrier (BBB), there will be Gd^{3+} extravasation, which will appear bright on T1-weighted imaging. Infectious, neoplastic, and inflammatory processes are typical causes of enhancing brain lesions

TABLE 10-1

Common Causes of Headaches Based on Location

Location of Pain	Neurologic Localization	Common Causes
Retro-orbital	Pain from optic nerve or retina irritation transmitted via the ophthalmic branch of the trigeminal nerve	Optic neuritis, temporal arteritis, migraine
Temple	Ophthalmic branch of trigeminal nerve innervates carotid artery for pain sensation	Temporal arteritis, carotid dissection, trigeminal neuralgia
Cheek	Maxillary branch of trigeminal nerve	Tooth abscess, trigeminal neuralgia
Jaw	Mandibular branch of trigeminal nerve	Temporomandibular joint (TMJ), tooth abscess, trigeminal neuralgia
Unilateral occiput	C2 dermatome, which innervates the vertebral artery	Vertebral artery dissection, occipital neuralgia, posterior fossa tumor
Ear	Complex—medial part innervated by trigeminal nerve, lateral part innervated by C2 dermatome; pain referred from trigeminal, glossopharyngeal, vagus, and facial nerve distributions	Middle ear infection, TMJ syndrome, trigeminal neuralgia
Neck	Meningeal irritation transmitted by C2 dermatome	SAH, meningitis
Vertex	Local meningeal stretching transmitted as dull pain by C2 dermatome	Brain tumor, elevated intracranial pressure, tension headache

and can cause headache through concomitant meningeal or vascular irritation. Diffusion-weighted imaging should be performed to assess for stroke. T2-weighted and fluid-attenuated inversion recovery (FLAIR) images assess for neoplastic, infectious, inflammatory, or ischemic processes and are the best studies to look for vasogenic edema. MR angiograms can assess the cerebral vasculature for aneurysm, dissection, or vascular malformations. MR venogram is used to determine the patency of the venous sinuses for evidence of venous sinus thrombosis. Other specialized MR-based studies can determine the direction or flow of cerebrospinal fluid within the ventricular system. These studies can be useful in the evaluation of patients with hydrocephalus, Arnold-Chiari malformation, and pseudotumor cerebri.

Assessment

In neurologic disease, assessment consists of anatomic or functional localization followed by the differential diagnosis. As discussed previously, headache localizes to the blood vessels, meninges, muscle, bone, and skin of the head and face. Table 10-1 shows the causes of common locations of head and face pain.

CLINICAL PEARL

Unlike the rest of neurology, the use of localization for etiologic identification of head pain is notoriously inaccurate. Therefore, Table 10.1 should be used as a source of clues to diagnosis rather than as a set of rules.

Tables 10-2 and 10-3 show common kinds of headache and the key aspects of diagnosis divided into primary and secondary headache syndromes. Primary headache syndromes are highly prevalent and account for one of the most common visits to the emergency room and primary care physician. Distinguishing between primary and secondary headache syndromes is important because it determines level of care (admission vs. outpatient care), level of acuity (emergency vs. nonemergent), prognosis, and chance of recurrence. Anyone with a new headache pattern should be evaluated and ruled out for a secondary headache syndrome before giving the diagnosis of a primary headache syndrome.

Secondary headache is a symptom of another disease process. The causes of secondary headache range from the relatively benign, such as toothache, to the severe, such as intracranial hemorrhage. There are many kinds of secondary headache, and Table 10-3 breaks them down by category.

Treatment

As with all medical diseases, treatment is directed at correcting the underlying abnormality as well as at providing symptomatic management. Table 10-4 lists

TABLE 10-2

Primary Headache Syndromes Based on the History, Exam, and Tests

Syndrome	Associated History and Symptoms	Exam Findings	Diagnostic Labs/Imaging
Migraine headache	Throbbing headache, nausea, vomiting, phonophobia, or photophobia.	Normal, or uncommonly with reversible focal neurologic findings	Labs and imaging usually normal
Tension headache	Bandlike pain around head, muscle aches, jaw clenching.	Usually none	Normal
Cluster headache	Unilateral lacrimation, runny nose, injected sclerae occurring several times daily for ~30 min to 2 hr at a time.	May have unilateral Horner's syndrome during attack	Normal
Paroxysmal hemicrania	<20-min bursts of unilateral head pain that cluster over about 24 hours. Attacks can cluster within weeks to months. Usually associated with autonomic symptoms.	None, or signs of autonomic activation (ptosis, lacrimation, scleral injection, rhinorrhea)	Normal
Hemicrania continua	Continuous unilateral migraine-like headache lasting days to weeks with intermittent worsening for minutes. Exacerbations can be associated with autonomic symptoms.	None, or signs of autonomic activation (ptosis, lacrimation, scleral injection, rhinorrhea)	Normal

TABLE 10-3

Secondary Headache Syndromes Based on the History, Exam, and Tests, and Divided by Category

Syndrome	Associated History and Symptoms	Exam Findings	Diagnostic Labs/Imaging
Vascular			
Subarachnoid hemorrhage	"Worst headache of life," neck pain and stiffness, photophobia and phonophobia	Diminished level of consciousness, focal neurologic deficits.	Head CT reveals subarachnoid blood, LP reveals RBCs and xanthochromia.
Intracerebral hemorrhage	Rapid onset of focal neurologic deficits: weakness, numbness, aphasia, ataxia	Elevated blood pressure, seizures, diminished level of consciousness, focal neurologic deficits.	Head CT reveals blood in brain parenchyma.
Epidural hemorrhage	Initial loss of consciousness, then recovery of consciousness with headache and a period of lucidity	Diminished level of consciousness, focal neurologic deficits.	Head CT reveals lentiform hematoma caused by laceration of middle meningeal artery.

(continued)

TABLE 10-3

Secondary Headache Syndromes Based on the History, Exam, and Tests, and Divided by Category (Continued)

Syndrome	Associated History and Symptoms	Exam Findings	Diagnostic Labs/Imaging
Vascular			
Subdural hemorrhage	Focal neurologic deficits, acute loss of consciousness, dementia if chronic	Seizures, focal neurologic deficits.	Head CT reveals crescent-shaped hematoma from laceration of bridging veins.
Ischemic stroke	Rarely causes headache (≤5%) but will have associated focal neurologic symptoms that develop abruptly	Focal neurologic deficits.	Head CT reveals hypodensity by 24 hours. Diffusion-weighted MRI reveals stroke as a hyperintensity within minutes.
Venous sinus thrombosis	Focal neurologic symptoms, especially visual loss, seizures	Papilledema, loss of visual fields, focal neurologic deficits, seizures.	T2-weighted MRI reveals flow voids in venous sinuses. MRV reveals filling abnormality. Gold standard is angiogram with venous phase.

Vertebral dissection	Pain radiating in neck, nausea, vomiting, vertigo, diplopia, dysarthria, dysphagia	Ipsilateral Horner's syndrome, cranial neuropathies, crossed exam findings consistent with brain stem infarction.	CT, MR, or conventional angiogram reveal false lumen within vertebral artery.
Carotid dissection	Pain radiating to temple, focal neurologic symptoms	Ipsilateral Horner's syndrome	CT, MR, or conventional angiogram reveal false lumen within carotid artery.
Arteriovenous malformation	Seizures, focal neurologic symptoms (weakness, numbness, language deficits)	Focal neurologic deficits. Bruit may be heard depending on location.	Angiogram or CTA demonstrates cluster of vessels usually with draining vein.
Infectious/Inflammatory			
Meningitis	Neck stiffness, fever, systemic infection, diminished level of consciousness	Pain on eye movement, nuchal rigidity, Brudzinski and Kernig signs. Some meningitides associated with rashes.	LP reveals elevated WBCs and protein. Glucose usually low in bacterial meningitis and normal in viral meningitis. Elevated monocytes usually associated with viral or tuberculosis (TB) infection. Elevated PMNs associated with bacterial infection.

(continued)

TABLE 10-3

Secondary Headache Syndromes Based on the History, Exam, and Tests, and Divided by Category (Continued)

Syndrome	Associated History and Symptoms	Exam Findings	Diagnostic Labs/Imaging
Infectious/Inflammatory			
Encephalitis	Seizures, focal neurologic deficits, confusion	Altered levels and content of consciousness. Focal neurologic deficits.	LP reveals elevated WBCs and protein. Glucose usually low in bacterial meningitis and normal in viral meningitis. Elevated monocytes usually associated with viral infection. Elevated PMNs associated with bacterial infection.
Brain abscess	Focal neurologic deficits	Papilledema, focal neurologic deficits, stigmata of other infections, such as HIV.	T2-weighted MRI reveals many with vasogenic edema; T1 with Gd^{3+} reveals rim of enhancement. LP will likely have elevated protein and monocytic pleocytosis if abscess wall is intact.

Sarcoidosis	Focal neurologic symptoms; look for symptoms in other organ systems, such as shortness of breath, cough, sinusitis	CSF pleocytosis, MRI T1 with Gd^{3+} reveals blood-brain barrier breakdown; hyperintensities on T2 MRI reveal acute and chronic lesions. Chest CT reveals hilar lymphadenopathy.
Lupus	Focal neurologic deficits	CSF pleocytosis, MRI T1 with Gd^{3+} reveals blood-brain barrier breakdown. Diffusion-weighted imaging reveals stroke.
Temporal arteritis	Fever, jaw claudication, temple pain, head and scalp allodynia, visual loss, generalized aches and malaise	ESR and CRP elevated but may be normal in 20%. Gold standard is temporal artery biopsy.
	Seizures, altered level of consciousness, or focal neurologic deficits to suggest recent stroke.	
	Loss of vision, decreased visual acuity, loss of color vision, weak temporal artery pulses, and thickened arteries.	
Optic neuritis	Sudden loss of visual acuity or color vision, pain behind eye especially with movement	Optical coherence tomography reveals thinned retinal layer. Visual evoked potentials reveal delayed responses in affected eye. MRI of brain and spinal cord should be performed to evaluate for MS.
	Loss of vision and color vision. Optic disk may appear normal or swollen.	

(continued)

TABLE 10-3

Secondary Headache Syndromes Based on the History, Exam, and Tests, and Divided by Category (Continued)

Syndrome	Associated History and Symptoms	Exam Findings	Diagnostic Labs/Imaging
Infectious/Inflammatory			
Trigeminal neuralgia	Stabbing electrical shocklike pains, which can be unilateral or bilateral	Usually normal	Angiography may reveal ectopic blood vessel that can irritate the trigeminal nerve.
Trauma			
Concussion	Recent trauma, loss of consciousness, memory loss, tinnitus, light sensitivity, blurred vision	If severe, seizures, diminished level of consciousness, pupil asymmetry, abnormal neuropsychologic testing (chronic).	Usually normal. Presence of subtle changes on MRI or PET is controversial.
Metabolic			
Hypoxia	Obesity, poor sleep with many arousals, smoking, alcoholism, morning headaches that improve	Obesity, clubbing, wheezing, may have low pulse oximetry reading, but may also be normal	Sleep study, pulse oximetry, arterial blood gas

Hypoglycemia	Diabetic on medications; may experience symptoms of sympathetic nervous system activation: sweating, tachycardia, nervousness	Diaphoretic, may have depressed level of consciousness or even focal neurologic deficits (stroke mimicker)	Basic metabolic panel or finger-stick glucose test
Carbon monoxide poisoning	Flu-like symptoms, depression, chest pain, shortness of breath	Hypertension, tachycardia, depressed level of consciousness. Chronically, dementia, parkinsonism, cortical blindness.	Elevated carboxyhemoglobin levels are diagnostic. Bilateral globus pallidus hyperintensities on T2 MRI.
Medications	Chronic daily headache or headaches at predictable times of day. May complain of other medication-specific side effects (constipation for narcotics)	Narcotics are most common offender—signaled by psychomotor slowing and miosis.	Toxicology screen, basic metabolic panel, arterial blood gas, outside medication records.

(continued)

TABLE 10-3

Secondary Headache Syndromes Based on the History, Exam, and Tests, and Divided by Category (Continued)

Syndrome	Associated History and Symptoms	Exam Findings	Diagnostic Labs/Imaging
Abnormalities of Intracranial Pressure			
Hydrocephalus (can be obstructive or nonobstructive)	If chronic, gradual worsening of cognition, gait, and urinary incontinence. If acute, depressed level of consciousness and herniation syndromes	Large head, cognition and gait abnormalities. Urinary incontinence. If acute, can lead to diminished level of consciousness or herniation.	Large ventricles on T2 or T1 MRI or noncontrast head CT. If severe, transependymal edema can be seen best on T2 MRI.
Pseudotumor cerebri (aka idiopathic intracranial hypertension)	Headaches worse in the morning, recent weight gain, visual changes, diplopia	Papilledema, extraocular motion abnormalities, visual field cuts, otherwise normal neurologic exam by definition.	May be normal, have small ventricles, or venous outflow obstruction on MRV or conventional venogram.

Congenital/Developmental

Arnold-Chiari malformation (downward displacement of cerebellar tonsils through the foramen magnum)	Intense throbbing in back of head, crania, diplopia, ataxia, tinnitus, dysphagia, dysarthria, numbness, especially on upper arms and torso, back pain	Cranial neuropathies, ataxia, evidence of syringomyelia (capelike distribution of numbness).	Cerebellar displacement best visualized on sagittal or coronal T1 or T2 MRI.
Dandy-Walker malformation (posterior fossa cyst formation, large fourth ventricle, absent cerebellar vermis)	Irritability, discoordination, difficulties walking, nausea and vomiting if intracranial pressure increases as a result	Large head and ataxia, papilledema, eye motion abnormalities, and breathing pattern problems when decompensated.	MRI or CT reveal malformation.
Low CSF pressure headache (can be owing to recent dural puncture, such as lumbar puncture, iatrogenic overdraining, such as through a shunt, or owing to traumatic CSF leak)	Headache worse with standing and better when lying down; tinnitus, neck pain.	If severe, can be associated with subdural hematoma, which can present with diminished level of consciousness, seizures, focal neurologic deficits.	T1 MRI with Gd^{3+} reveals diffuse pachymeningeal enhancement best observed in coronal views.

(continued)

TABLE 10-3

Secondary Headache Syndromes Based on the History, Exam, and Tests, and Divided by Category (Continued)

Syndrome	Associated History and Symptoms	Exam Findings	Diagnostic Labs/Imaging
Neoplastic			
Brain tumors	Gradual onset of focal neurologic deficits, headaches worst in a.m.	Papilledema, seizures, focal neurologic deficits, signs of systemic illness.	CT with contrast and T1 MRI with contrast demonstrate different patterns of enhancement that vary based on the tumor. T2 MRI and noncontrast CT show vasogenic edema.
Dental Issues			
Toothache	Tooth sensitivity to normal stimuli, such as hot and cold	Pain on palpation. Abscess may cause mass effect on tooth.	Dental films may show abscess or cavity.
Temporomandibular joint (TMJ) syndrome	Ear pain, jaw muscle pain and fatigue, clicking with opening of jaw	Jaw muscle trigger points and crepitus over TMJ.	Tooth radiographs to exclude tooth pathology as cause.

TABLE 10-4

Treatment of Primary and Secondary Headache Syndromes

Syndrome	Acute Treatment	Ongoing Treatment
Primary Headache Syndromes		
Migraine headache	Triptans, NSAIDs, migraine cocktail (steroids, antiemetic, NSAIDs, magnesium sulfate given IV at the same time), DHE.	Migraine prophylaxis (beta-blockers, calcium channel blockers, antidepressants, antiepileptics).
Tension headache	NSAIDs, perhaps Tylenol	Identify and eliminate triggers, such as stress, fatigue, ergonomic stresses.
Cluster headache	Nasal cannula O_2	
Paroxysmal hemicrania	Indomethacin. Prophylaxis against peptic disease is important.	Usually remit, but chronic low-dose indomethacin may be required.
Hemicrania continua	Indomethacin. Prophylaxis against peptic disease is important.	Indomethacin is usually required chronically.
Secondary Headache Syndromes		
Vascular		
Subarachnoid hemorrhage	Clipping or coiling of aneurysm by neurosurgery.	May have migraines, seizures, and neurologic disability from stroke owing to vasospasm as long-term complications.

(continued)

TABLE 10-4

Treatment of Primary and Secondary Headache Syndromes (Continued)

Syndrome	Acute Treatment	Ongoing Treatment
Secondary Headache Syndromes		
Vascular		
Intracerebral hemorrhage	Lower blood pressure, correct coagulopathies, and manage elevated intracranial pressure.	Identify and eliminate risk factors wherever possible, such as hypertension, cocaine use. May have migraines, seizures, and neurologic disability as long-term complications.
Epidural hemorrhage	Hemorrhage evacuation by neurosurgery.	May have migraines, seizures, and rebleeding as long-term complications.
Subdural hemorrhage	Hemorrhage evacuation by neurosurgery.	May have migraines, seizures, and rebleeding as long-term complications.
Ischemic stroke	Determine if patient is a candidate for thrombolytics, call neurology, give aspirin, allow blood pressure to run higher to optimize perfusion, manage intracranial hypertension if applicable.	May have migraines, seizures, and neurologic disability as long-term complications.

TABLE 10-4

Treatment of Primary and Secondary Headache Syndromes (Continued)

Syndrome	Acute Treatment	Ongoing Treatment
Secondary Headache Syndromes		
Venous sinus thrombosis	Anticoagulation with unfractionated heparin to prevent extension of the thrombus.	Anticoagulation for 3–6 months with oral warfarin. Identify and exclude risk factors if possible, including dehydration, pregnancy, hormone replacement therapy, hypercoagulable states owing to autoimmune disease or cancer.
Vertebral dissection	Anticoagulation with unfractionated heparin to prevent embolic stroke from thrombus within the dissection.	Anticoagulation for 3–6 months with oral warfarin.
Carotid dissections	Anticoagulation with unfractionated heparin to prevent embolic stroke from thrombus within the dissection. If stroke involves more than 1/3 of the cerebral hemisphere, anticoagulation is relatively contraindicated.	Anticoagulation for 3–6 months with oral warfarin.
Arteriovenous malformation (AVM)	Craniotomy or endovascular surgery by neurosurgery.	May have migraines, seizures, and neurologic disability as long-term complications, especially if the AVM ruptured.

(continued)

TABLE 10-4

Treatment of Primary and Secondary Headache Syndromes (Continued)

Syndrome	Acute Treatment	Ongoing Treatment
Secondary Headache Syndromes		
Infectious/inflammatory		
Meningitis	Ceftriaxone, vancomycin, ampicillin, and acyclovir until sensitivities known. Four days of dexamethasone if pneumococcus is offending bacteria. Consider tuberculosis treatment if the patient has tuberculosis exposure or if the CSF glucose is very low and monocytes predominate.	May have migraines, seizures, hydrocephalus as long-term complications.
Encephalitis	Ceftriaxone, vancomycin, ampicillin, and acyclovir until sensitivities known. If HIV positive, immune reconstitution is imperative.	May have migraines, seizures, hydrocephalus as long-term complications.
Brain abscess	Broad-spectrum antibiotics to cover both aerobic and anaerobic bacteria. If HIV positive, consider treatment for toxoplasmosis.	May have migraines, seizures, hydrocephalus as long-term complications.

TABLE 10-4

Treatment of Primary and Secondary Headache Syndromes (Continued)

Syndrome	Acute Treatment	Ongoing Treatment
Secondary Headache Syndromes		
Sarcoidosis	Pulse IV steroid treatment if severe with focal neurologic deficits.	Chronic immunosuppression.
Lupus	Pulse IV steroid treatment if severe with focal neurologic deficits.	Chronic immunosuppression
Temporal arteritis	Pulse IV steroid treatment. If vision is threatened, do not delay treatment. NSAIDs can also provide pain relief.	Immunosuppression for at least 1 year.
Optic neuritis	Pulse IV steroid treatment with 11-day taper with oral prednisone.	Evaluation for MS and start MS disease-modifying therapy if appropriate.
Trigeminal Neuralgia	Cold packs, anti-epileptics (carbamazepine and phenytoin are effective within hours)	Surgical microvascular decompression
Trauma		
Concussion	Manage seizures and headaches.	Manage migraines and depression.

(continued)

TABLE 10-4

Treatment of Primary and Secondary Headache Syndromes (Continued)

Syndrome	Acute Treatment	Ongoing Treatment
Secondary Headache Syndromes		
Metabolic		
Hypoxia	Oxygen per nasal cannula.	Identify cause and treat. If obstructive sleep apnea, lose weight and institute continuous positive airway pressure at night.
Hypoglycemia	Ampule of IV dextrose and/or encourage PO intake.	Identify cause and avoid agents that induce hypoglycemia.
Carbon monoxide poisoning	Hyperbaric oxygen	Eliminate cause.
Medications	Medication antidote and/or activated charcoal.	Medication organization systems, such as a pillbox. Primary care provider involvement.
Abnormalities of Intracranial Pressure		
Hydrocephalus	Carbonic anhydrase inhibitors, such as acetazolamide and topiramate, reduce CSF production. Lumbar puncture or catheter drainage if communicating hydrocephalus.	Surgically placed shunt or third ventriculostomy.

TABLE 10-4

Treatment of Primary and Secondary Headache Syndromes (Continued)

Syndrome	Acute Treatment	Ongoing Treatment
Secondary Headache Syndromes		
Pseudotumor cerebri	Carbonic anhydrase inhibitors, such as acetazolamide and topiramate, reduce CSF production. Lumbar puncture or catheter drainage.	Pain control. About 2/3 remit spontaneously. If severe and vision is threatened, surgically placed shunt.
Arnold-Chiari malformation	Shunt placement if hydrocephalus occurs. No lumbar procedures.	Shunt placement if hydrocephalus occurs. No lumbar procedures.
Dandy-Walker malformation	Shunt placement or cyst drainage if symptoms are severe.	Shunt placement or cyst drainage if symptoms are severe.
Low CSF pressure headache	IV fluids and caffeine. Blood patch placed by anesthesiology where venous blood is injected into epidural space.	
Neoplastic		
Brain tumors	Seizure control. Corticosteroids to reduce inflammation and mass effect only if impending herniation or severe disability. Steroids can make the diagnosis of certain tumors impossible, such as lymphoma.	Surgery for debulking and pathologic diagnosis. Chemotherapy and radiation depending on specific tumor.

(continued)

TABLE 10-4
Treatment of Primary and Secondary Headache Syndromes (Continued)

Syndrome	Acute Treatment	Ongoing Treatment
Secondary Headache Syndromes		
Dental Issues		
Toothache	Root canal or cavity treatment.	Dental care.
TMJ syndrome	NSAIDs or jaw muscle massage or stretching.	Orthodontics, dental care, bite guard for bruxism.

NSAIDs, nonsteroidal anti-inflammatory drugs; DHE, dihydroergotamine; MS, multiple sclerosis; PO, by mouth.

the common therapies for primary headache syndromes and secondary headaches syndromes divided into acute and ongoing treatments.

EXTENDED INHOSPITAL MANAGEMENT

The initial workup focuses on ruling out life-threatening emergencies. Once those disorders are ruled out, the extended workup is individually tailored to the specific condition. Some diseases are difficult to diagnose and require intensive workup, such as vasculitis. Other diseases are easily diagnosed but are difficult to treat, such as intractable migraines.

DISPOSITION
Discharge Goals

Ideally, when the patient is discharged, the headache is resolved and the underlying abnormality that led to the headache is corrected. Practically, there are two goals for patients admitted for headache:

1. Rule out life-threatening conditions.
2. Arrive at a diagnosis and treatment plan that will lead to the resolution of headache and the underlying abnormality.

It may take time for headaches associated with many neurologic diseases to resolve, and patients may still require significant symptomatic therapy when they are discharged to rehabilitation. In every case, there must be a treatment plan in place by discharge that will eventually lead to resolution of headache and the underlying condition if known.

Outpatient Care

Conditions that are generally treated on an outpatient basis are the following:

- Migraine headaches (and cluster headaches)
- Tension headaches
- Chronic daily headache
- Pseudotumor cerebri

However, there are occasions when patient with these conditions may require intensive inpatient therapy.

Follow-up for patients who developed headache from an acute intracranial event, such as a hemorrhage or an infection, should be arranged with an outpatient neurologist prior to discharge to ensure that the underlying condition is resolved or is resolving and that the symptoms are adequately managed at home.

 WHAT YOU NEED TO REMEMBER

- Primary headache syndromes are due to irritation of nerve endings in the blood vessels, meninges, muscle, bone, and skin of the head and face.
- Secondary headaches are caused by an underlying condition. These may be acute, such as an intracranial hemorrhage, or a chronic condition, such as lupus.
- Any new acute headache must be worked up either on an inpatient or outpatient basis depending on the suspected cause.
- An urgent head CT to rule out a life-threatening condition should be obtained for patients presenting to the emergency room with an acute new headache.
- Inpatient workup may require more invasive testing to make a diagnosis.
- Discharge does not always depend on complete resolution of headache symptoms, but a treatment plan must be in place and a follow-up evaluation arranged.

SUGGESTED READINGS

Silberstein SD, Lipton RB, Dodick DW, eds. *Wolff's Headache and Other Head Pain.* 8th Ed. New York: Oxford University Press, USA, 2007.

11

Speech, Language, and Cognition

A 71-year-old, right-handed man with a history of atrial fibrillation and alcohol abuse was found by family on the floor of his home. He was not moving the right side of his body, he was not speaking, and he appeared confused. The duration of symptoms was unknown, but he had been seen interacting normally 48 hours earlier.

OVERVIEW

Definition and Pathophysiology

The ability to create sounds with the intent to communicate requires a highly coordinated interplay between the speech, language, and higher-order cognitive centers of the brain. Speech is the ability to vocalize by coordinating the muscles that control the vocal apparatus—it is the mechanical aspect of oral communication. Language, on the other hand, refers to symbolic communication made possible by central processing. Language is the software program that is output through the speech hardware. For example, if you want to say, "I want to do well on my neurology clerkship," you must first encode the sentence through your language centers before you speak this sentence using your speech apparatus.

Thus, any patient who cannot communicate effectively may have pathology affecting at least one of these components. Because speech, language, and cognition are subserved by different parts of the nervous system, it is important to determine which aspect is affected so that you can provide the correct diagnosis and intervention.

Speech requires two distinct components: phonation and articulation. Phonation is the ability to produce sound and requires the respiratory musculature, which is innervated by the phrenic nerve, and it requires the larynx, which is innervated by the recurrent laryngeal nerve. Problems with phonation can result from damage to any of these structures. Articulation is the ability to produce precise vocal expressions and requires the pharynx, tongue, lips, and facial muscles, all of which are innervated by cranial nerves.

The job of language is to name objects and ideas. Language processes are lateralized to the left cerebral hemisphere in most people. Language content undergoes preliminary decoding in the Wernicke area, which is located in the superior temporal lobe. Information then travels from Wernicke' area through the arcuate fasciculus to Broca's area, which initiates a motor output to pronounce words. This will be more fully discussed later in the chapter when we discuss the assessment.

CLINICAL PEARL

Approximately 25% of left-handed individuals will lateralize their language centers to the right cerebral hemisphere or share it between both hemispheres.

Even if the language and speech pathways are intact, communication may be nonsensical because of a disruption of cognition. Thinking is the most complex task that humans perform and is poorly understood. However, it is clear that the frontal lobes and other association areas in the parietal cortices are integral in producing coherent thought processes. The decline of cognitive ability is called dementia. Dementia can be caused by several conditions, but they all lead to the same disabilities: difficulty with higher thinking, forming memories, making calculations, and recognizing places and faces.

Dementias are divided into two classes: cortical and subcortical. Cortical dementias cause dysfunction with the cerebral cortex, which leads to memory impairment, speech/language problems, and personality change. The classic cortical dementia is Alzheimer's disease. Subcortical dementias cause dysfunction of the deeper structures of the brain, including the white matter and basal ganglia. Subcortical dementias are defined by motor involvement in the form of slowing. The classic subcortical dementias are multi-infarct dementia and Parkinson disease.

Epidemiology

Dementia affects up to 10% of the population of the United States and affects up to 24% of the elderly older than 85 years of age. It is the most common cause of institutionalization in this age group and is associated with higher mortality regardless of the cause of death. In other words, when a person with dementia has a myocardial infarction, he or she is more likely to die than is an individual without dementia. This is most likely caused by poor understanding and communication, which leads to delayed care.

ACUTE MANAGEMENT AND WORKUP

The spectrum of conditions that lead to problems with speech, language, and cognitive problems range from the mild sore throat to a devastating stroke. All patients with acute difficulty in speech, language, and cognition, regardless of past medical history, should be evaluated quickly to rule out life-threatening conditions. Remember, even patients with Alzheimer's dementia should still be evaluated and treated for an acute stroke.

The First 15 Minutes

The first 15 minutes in the evaluation of a patient with speech and language problems or with problems with cognition is to stabilize your patient and gather data together from as many sources as possible to determine the history of the present illness.

Initial Assessment

Look at the patient. Is he awake and alert or drowsy? Is the patient protecting his airway or is he having trouble clearing his secretions? Is the patient's face symmetric or drooping? Is the patient moving all of his limbs or is he hemiparetic? Quickly get a sense of your patient's general condition and make sure the ABCs (airway, breathing, circulation) are controlled.

After stabilizing the patient, the next step is to narrow down the problem from "not speaking" to dysarthria (problem with speech), dysphasia (problem with language), or dementia (problem with cognition). In the acute setting, this may be difficult because the patient will not be able to tell you what is wrong. You have to use clues from the family members who brought him to the emergency department (ED) and from your physical exam.

Patients with acute presentations of dysarthria should be able to follow all commands and communicate with you in some way, either by writing or talking, albeit with difficulty. Look at the patient's mouth, throat, neck, and chest to rule out a mechanical issue. For example, in Bell's palsy, paresis of the cheek on one side of the face will lead to dysarthria. Patients with acute presentations of dysphasia will either have difficulty understanding language, producing language, or both. Patients with acute presentations of dementia are rare and usually have a history of chronic dementia with a superimposed metabolic derangement, such as urinary tract infection or pneumonia.

Quickly decide what speech, language, or cognitive problem your patient has and convey your concerns to your senior resident.

Admission Criteria and Level of Care Criteria

Any patient with an acute onset of disease that could be life threatening should be admitted, worked up, and treated. Such diseases include acute stroke, seizures, infection, trauma, and worsening of neoplastic processes. Any chronic disease that has progressed to a point that the patient's airway or ability to take care of himself is affected should also be admitted. Such diseases include amyotrophic lateral sclerosis (ALS), myasthenia gravis, chronic dementia, and neoplastic processes. Finally, any patient who is a threat to himself or others because of the psychological complications of his neurologic illness should also be admitted.

The First 24 Hours

The first 24 hours of workup will focus on localizing the lesion and making the diagnosis. Toward this goal, the history and physical exam are critical in narrowing your differential diagnosis, and the labs and imaging studies you order are useful in confirming your diagnosis.

History

There are three key aspects of the history. First, find out when the problem with speech, language, and/or cognition began, how it has changed, and the speed with which it has progressed. Second, narrow down more specifically which aspect of speech, language, and/or cognition has been affected. Third, sort out if any other symptoms are present and their temporal relationship with the speech, language, and/or cognition pathology. Finally, once you ascertain these key history findings, assess any risk factors important in the development of certain pathologies, including past medical history, tobacco use, alcohol use, illicit substance use, and the family history.

The items below include the questions you will need to ask, the actions you will need to take, and patient care aspects you will need to consider when you gather the patient's history.

- *Time course of the disorder.* Ask the patient's family about the time course of this particular problem. If the family insists that your patient was totally normal before the onset of this problem, make sure you document the time the patient was last seen normal by someone. For example, if the patient woke up dysphasic but was seen normal by his wife going to bed last night, the time last seen normal was last night. The acute change could have theoretically occurred anytime during the night. Also ask if the symptoms have been getting worse, getting better, or have stayed the same. A transient, reversible loss of speech/language/cognition carries a different differential diagnosis.

  For more chronic problems, such as dementia, ask about the days leading up to the acute change. Find out if there were symptoms present before this acute presentation that would provide clues to this diagnosis. For example, family may tell you that your patient has been complaining of burning with urination for the past 3 days, which suggests a urinary tract infection. When documenting the time course of a chronic disorder, especially dementia, it is very helpful to ask about specific tasks such as balancing checkbooks and cooking.

- *Narrowing down the problem.* As opposed to your initial 15-minute assessment, now you have plenty of time to explore the actual problem. Your patient presented "not talking" but that could be because of speech, language, or cognitive problems, or any combination of these.

  - *Speech difficulties.* Problems with speech should not affect communication. Your patient should certainly be able to understand you and follow your commands. If the patient has speech problems, he should be able to try to talk, even if the resulting speech is muffled, garbled, or hypophonic. Writing should be intact. Ask the family about your patient's ability to understand them and communicate with them.

- *Language difficulties.* Language difficulty could be owing to either poor understanding or poor production of language. Ask the patient or family about the specific problems the patient had with language, and ask for examples.
- *Cognitive difficulties.* Cognitive problems can range from minor memory difficulties to frank dementia. Ask what specific difficulties the patient has paying close attention to short- and long-term memory, following directions, getting lost, paying attention. Make sure you get a sense for the duration of involvement. The vast majority of cognitive problems are not acute.

- *Associated pathologies.* Many patients with speech, language, or cognitive problems have had difficulties in these areas previously and now have a superimposed difficulty caused by a systemic abnormality such as infection. This phenomenon is called *neurologic reserve* and is described in more detail in Chapter 3, Altered Mental Status. In brief, neurologic reserve is the ability of the brain to buffer against systemic abnormality. The classic example that is relevant to cognitive problems is a well-adjusted Alzheimer's patient who develops a urinary tract infection. In this case, the patient's neurologic reserve is poor because of Alzheimer's disease and is susceptible to acute decline owing to a systemic metabolic disturbance from a urinary tract infection. Thus, it is important to collect information about associated issues that may be related. Ask about symptoms related to urination, as well as to the respiratory, cardiac, and hematologic systems.

Physical Examination

The physical examination should evaluate phonation, articulation, language, and cognition separately.

- *Phonation.* The initial examination of phonation involves assessing spontaneous speech during conversation when taking the patient's history.
  - Assess whether the patient's speech is present and, if so, if it is breathy or hoarse.
  - Investigate whether there are other signs that suggest possible phonation pathology, such as rapid, shallow, or labored breathing; audible, breathy inspiration; and inhalation stridor.
- *Articulation.* The initial examination of articulation involves assessing spontaneous speech during conversation when taking the patient's history.

- Further special testing of speech involves repetition of test words and phrases, such as "la, la, la," "ma, ma, ma," "ga, ga, ga." These sounds test the lingual, labial, and guttural sounds, respectively.
- You can also have the patient read a paragraph from a magazine or pamphlet. Listen carefully to how the speech sounds:
  - Flaccid dysarthria. Slurred speech, difficulty with labial consonants, and a nasal quality often point to a lower motor neuron problem such as Guillain-Barré, or myasthenia gravis.
  - Spastic dysarthria. This is a harsh, low-pitched, slow, and monotonous verbal output that sounds strained. It often points to upper motor neuron lesions from strokes or ALS.
  - Ataxic dysarthria. Slow and slurred speech with sudden uncontrolled alteration in the loudness of the voice can suggest cerebellar diseases, such as those seen in alcoholism.
  - Hypokinetic dysarthria. Slow and usually hypophonic speech can be seen in parkinsonism.
- Any patient with suspected dysarthria should have a detailed cranial nerve examination that looks especially at the mouth, palate, pharynx, and tongue.
- *Language.* You should have the patient perform four tasks that will help to localize the pathology:
  1. First, ask the patient to name objects; you can start simply, providing objects such as a pen and wristwatch and progressing to more uncommon objects for the patient, such as stethoscope.
  2. Second, ask the patient to repeat a phrase perfectly, such as "no ifs, ands, or buts." Note that repetition is affected by lesions in the perisylvian zone.
  3. Third, assess the patient's fluency in his ability to produce words.
  4. Fourth, assess comprehension by asking the patient to perform both a one-step task (e.g., closing his eyes) and a multistep task (e.g., taking his left thumb and touching it to his right ear). The ability to perform these tasks gives clues as to the location of the pathology: Figure 11-1 shows the algorithm for localizing aphasia.
- *Cognition.* Cognition is difficult to completely test in a brief hospital encounter and requires neuropsychometric testing for completeness. However, your brief encounter as well as directed questions can give insight into the patient's cognition. For example, you can test the patient's memory by asking him to repeat the names of three objects (e.g., apple, wristwatch, and dragon) immediately and at 5 minutes. The complete Mini-Mental Status Exam described in Chapter 1, Localization and the Neurologic Exam, is a quick and useful test of cognition and orientation. You can also test the patient's judgment by asking questions like, "What would you do if you were stranded in an airport without any acquaintances and only $1?" You can test abstractions by asking questions like, "In what way are a painting and music alike?"

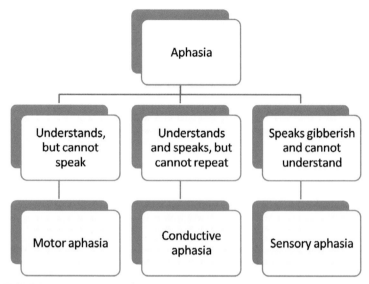

FIGURE 11-1: Algorithm for testing aphasia. If language output is compromised but understanding is intact, the diagnosis is *motor aphasia*. If understanding is compromised but language production is intact (although usually gibberish), the diagnosis is *sensory aphasia*. If only repetition is compromised, the diagnosis is *conductive aphasia*.

Labs and Tests to Consider

Based on your history and neurologic exam, you should have a sense for the type of testing needed to make a diagnosis. It is not necessary to send for all the labs listed in this section for every patient with speech, language, and/or cognitive disorders. In general, labs are useful in ruling out general systemic abnormalities whereas imaging is better for suspected primary central nervous system (CNS) pathologies.

Key Diagnostic Labs and Tests

Labs are not very helpful in diagnosing a primary neurologic disorder that causes speech, language, and cognitive disorders. One exception is the diagnosis of a focal cortical abscess from a spinal tap. However, as mentioned previously, common systemic abnormalities, such as pneumonia, urinary tract infections, and medication toxicities, can cause neurologic problems in patients with poor neurologic reserve. Table 11-1 lists lab tests to consider that focus on ruling out a superimposed metabolic abnormality in patients with poor neurologic reserve.

TABLE 11-1
Key Laboratory Tests and Rationales for Testing

Test	Rationale
Heme-8 with differential	Rule out leukocytosis.
Basic metabolic panel	Rule out evidence of metabolic dysfunction such as ARF, uremia, or an electrolyte imbalance, such as hyponatremia.
Specific drug levels	E.g. phenytoin, lithium.
Ethanol	Rule out alcohol intoxication.
Urine toxicity	Rule out toxic ingestion.
Urinalysis	Rule out UTI.
Blood/urine cultures	If infection is suspected.
Lumbar puncture	Lumbar puncture should be performed after head imaging if infection or demyelinating disease is suspected.

ARF, acute renal failure; UTI, urinary tract infection.

Imaging and Ancillary Testing

In contrast to lab testing, imaging of the brain is extremely useful in ruling out a primary neurologic pathology that causes speech, language, and cognitive disorders. The key diagnostic tests listed in Table 11-2 focus on ruling out a CNS pathology.

Assessment

The assessment is the part of the workup that synthesizes your thoughts about the history, the physical exam, lab tests, and imaging into a thoughtful review and judgment of the problem. For all neurologic patients, including those with speech, language, and cognitive disorders, the assessment consists of three major sections:

- *A succinct, summary sentence that includes the most important aspects of the history, physical exam, and tests.* Summarize the patient case in two or three sentences that include the important elements of the history, physical exam, and findings on testing that support your conclusion.
- *Localization.* Based on your workup of what the actual problem is—dysphonia, dysarthria, dysphasia/aphasia, or cognitive problems—localization

TABLE 11-2

Key Imaging Tests and Rationales for Testing

Test	Rationale
Noncontrast head computed tomography (CT)	Rule out intracranial hemorrhage from stroke or subarachnoid hemorrhage, subdural hemorrhage from trauma, previous strokes, and hydrocephalus.
Magnetic resonance imaging (MRI) of head	MRI of the brain with and without contrast is useful in determining if an acute stroke is present. MRI can also be helpful in delineating other potential pathologies including neoplastic processes, infections, and some degenerative diseases.
Electrophysiologic testing including electroencephalogram (EEG) and electromyogram (EMG)/nerve conduction study (NCS)	An EEG can be helpful if seizures are suspected. EMG and NCS can assist in the diagnosis of speech pathology from myasthenia gravis or ALS.
Neuropsychologic testing	Numerous tests beyond the scope of this chapter provide valuable information about cognitive function. These can be especially useful in the context of a patient with primary progressive aphasia or dementia.
Other	Laryngoscopy, CT of the face, and diaphragmatic fluoroscopy can be helpful in the diagnosis of peripheral causes of speech disorders.

starts with deciding between neurologic and nonneurologic causes. Among neurologic causes, try to narrow down the location of the lesion between the peripheral and the central nervous systems and then to the precise structure, cortex, or nerve involved.

• *Etiology*. Below are some of the more common causes of speech/language/cognitive problems. Following each of these causes are a series of questions to pose to yourself about the patient's history and physical that would support that cause:

  • Stroke. When was the patient last seen normal? Are there any associated symptoms, including weakness or sensory changes? What side of the body is affected? Is there associated ataxia or nystagmus?

  • Seizures. What was the time of onset? How long did the seizure last? Has this ever happened before? Is the patient on any antiepileptic medications? Does the patient drink alcohol?

  • Dementia. Has the patient been diagnosed with dementia in the past? How is the patient's memory? Does the patient balance his own checkbook? Does the patient drive? Have the patient's symptoms progressed?

  • Delirium. Is there a waxing and waning quality to the patient's level of consciousness? Does he have any risk factors for delirium?

  • Neoplasm. Does the patient have any risk factors for malignancy? Has the patient had any weight loss, fevers, or chills?

  • Infection. Does the patient have any fevers or chills? Does the patient have a stiff neck?

Table 11-3 lists the differential diagnoses for each category of impairment.

Treatment

The management of speech, language, and/or cognition pathology is twofold. First, one must initially treat the underlying disease causing the pathology. Most emergently, any patient with a suspected stroke should be admitted, worked up, and treated per stroke guidelines with the possibility of tissue plasminogen activator (tPA), especially if the patient presents within the 3- to 6-hour time window for thrombolysis. Unfortunately, in some cases (for example, with dementia), there may be no treatment other than supportive care. Second, one can provide therapy for regaining what has been lost.

All patients with speech, language, and/or cognition pathology should be seen by a speech pathologist who can help diagnose and treat the problem. In the case of dysphonia and dysarthria, the speech pathologist can determine a patient's eating safety. If the anatomy designed to protect the airway is too damaged, then a patient may aspirate and should remain NPO (nothing by mouth) or have a feeding tube placed until he is able to eat safely. A speech pathologist can also provide therapy and ways to optimize speech function. For example, physical tools may improve expression, particularly among global aphasics. One approach is to attach the weak right arm of a

TABLE 11-3
Differential Diagnoses of Speech, Language, and Cognitive Diseases

Dysphonia	Dysarthria	Dysphasia/Aphasia	Cognitive
Essential tremor	Stroke	Stroke	Primary dementia—e.g., Alzheimer's, frontotemporal dementia
	Neurodegenerative disorders—e.g., ALS, Parkinson's disease	Dementia	Delirium
Recurrent laryngeal nerve paresis	Multiple sclerosis	Infection	Multi-infarct (or vascular) dementia
Vocal cord nodules or polyps	Parkinson's disease	Neoplasm	Prion disease
Inflammation of the vocal cord (e.g., gastrointestinal [GI] reflux)	Lesions of cranial nerves—e.g., Lyme disease, sarcoid	Seizures	Alcohol-induced dementia (Korsakoff disease)
Neoplasm	Myasthenia gravis	Primary progressive aphasia	Psychiatric disease—e.g., mood disorders, schizophrenia
Infection of the vocal cord	Guillain-Barré	—	—
Trauma	Drug induced dysarthria	—	—
	Cerebellar diseases	—	—

patient with global aphasia to a device that grips a pen and permits it to smoothly glide over a sheet of paper, through the patient's voluntary propulsion at the shoulder. Surprisingly, this may allow crudely executed writing that is nonetheless more accurate at naming and dictation tasks than that accomplished by the nonparetic arm.

Finally, treatment should also address goals of care and identify limiting factors so that the patient, the patient's family, and the care provider understand the expected outcome and the duration of therapy.

EXTENDED INHOSPITAL MANAGEMENT

Inpatient workup for stroke is focused on finding the cause of the stroke to prevent a recurrence. Toward that end, carotid Dopplers and echocardiogram are done along with a series of typical stroke labs, such as cholesterol levels and thyroid function studies, that will help you stratify risk and reduce the chance for another stroke. If the patient's stroke workup is negative, consider the other causes listed in Table 11-3 and obtain the necessary tests to rule out each diagnosis.

DISPOSITION

Discharge Goals

There are three major discharge goals for patients with speech, language, and cognitive problems:

1. *Correction of the problem that caused the dysfunction.* In the case of an ischemic stroke, rehabilitation is the key treatment for improvement. Seizures respond to antiepileptic medications, Parkinson's disease to L-dopa, and so on.
2. *Prevention of recurrence of the problem and prevention of exacerbation.* These are accomplished by maintaining the patient's optimum neurologic health and addressing specific issues, such as carotid stenosis, that may lead to stroke recurrence.
3. *Establishing the level of care.* In certain patient populations, including the elderly and disabled, special consideration should be paid to the level of care. The family should be involved in discussions of nursing home care or other living arrangements, especially in cases of progressive dementing neurodegenerative diseases such as Alzheimer's disease.

CLINICAL PEARL

Hospice care is reserved for patients with terminal conditions and usually requires a Do Not Resuscitate (DNR)/Do Not Intubate (DNI) status.

Outpatient Care

All patients discharged with speech, language, and cognitive problems need follow-up after discharge, which should be arranged *before* the patient leaves the hospital. If the cause was determined to be primarily neurologic, such as seizures, follow-up should be arranged with a neurologist. If the cause was determined to be primarily medical, such as a urinary tract infection, follow-up should be arranged with the primary care physician.

WHAT YOU NEED TO REMEMBER

- The ability to create sounds with the intent to communicate requires a highly coordinated interplay between the speech, language, and higher-order cognitive centers of the brain.
- The spectrum of conditions that lead to problems with speech, language, and cognitive problems range from the mild sore throat to a devastating stroke. All patients with acute difficulty in speech, language, and cognition, regardless of past medical history, should be evaluated quickly to rule out life-threatening conditions.
- There are three key aspects of the workup for speech, language, and cognitive disorders: (i) the time course and progression of the disorder; (ii) the specific dysfunction of speech, language, and/or cognition; and (iii) identification of other signs and symptoms.
- The major types of aphasia are Wernicke's, sensory, motor, and Broca's aphasia. The most common causes of aphasia are stroke, degenerative disease, and tumors.
- The major types of dementia are cortical and subcortical. The most common cause of cortical dementia is Alzheimer's disease, and the most common cause of subcortical dementia is multi-infarct dementia. Parkinson's disease also leads to subcortical dementia.
- The workup usually involves imaging by MRI.
- Treatment depends on the specific cause.

SUGGESTED READINGS

Brazis PW, Masdeau JC, Biller J. *Localization in Clinical Neurology*. 6th Ed. Philadelphia: Lippincott Williams & Wilkins, 2006.

Ingram JCL. *Neurolinguistics: An Introduction to Spoken Language Processing and its Disorders*. Cambridge, UK: Cambridge University Press, 2007.

Patten JP. *Neurological Differential Diagnosis*. 2nd Ed. New York: Springer, 1998.

Mood Disorders

THE PATIENT ENCOUNTER

A 27-year-old woman presents to the emergency room and reports a 2-week history of low mood and suicidal ideation with a plan to overdose on medications.

OVERVIEW

Definition and Pathophysiology

Mood disorders are diseases that produce episodic fluctuations in mood and include major depressive disorder, bipolar disorder type I, bipolar disorder type II, substance-induced mood disorders, and adjustment disorder (Table 12-1). The episodes should last for a minimum of 2 weeks to classify as a major depressive disorder and 1 week to classify as a manic episode. If the patient does not fulfill the entire *Diagnostic Statistical Manual of Mental Disorders* (DSM) IV criteria for a particular episode or there is insufficient data to make a diagnosis, consider the diagnoses *depression not otherwise specified* or *mood disorders not otherwise specified*.

CLINICAL PEARL

Note that any patient who attempts suicide automatically receives the diagnosis of depression.

Research into the biologic mechanism underlying mood disorders has focused on the balance of biogenic amines: serotonin, norepinephrine, dopamine, histamine, and acetylcholine. Current theory holds that depression is caused by a decrease or dysregulation of these amines whereas mania is caused by excessive release.

Epidemiology

At any time, up to 9% of women and up to 3% of men in the United States meet clinical criteria for depression. Over a lifetime, 12% of men and 25% of women can expect to become depressed at some point. However, only 25% of depressed people ever seek treatment and most are treated by their

TABLE 12-1
Types of Mood Disorders

Mood Disorder	Description
Major depressive disorder	Typical depressive feelings associated with at least four of the following: sleep disturbance, appetite change, loss of interest, decreased energy, excessive guilt, concentration difficulty, psychomotor retardation, or suicidal ideation
Bipolar disorder, type I	Mania characterized by euphoria, grandiosity, being energetic, being distractible, having racing thoughts, having pressured speech and irritability; usually alternates with major depressive episodes.
Bipolar disorder, type II	Hypomania defined by mania that is *not* grossly incapacitating; may be associated with major depressive episodes.
Substance-induced mood disorders	Depression or mania only in the setting of intoxication or withdrawal from drugs or medications
Adjustment disorder	Sadness or anxiety caused by a recent event in life, such as illness or divorce. The stressor could be a single event or an ongoing issue.

primary care physicians. Bipolar disorders are rarer but still affect 1% of adults in the United States. Loss of a parent before age 15 has been associated with depression later in life.

ACUTE MANAGEMENT AND WORKUP

Up to 15% of depressed patients successfully commit suicide. Most of those patients will attempt suicide by prescription medication overdose. In addition to suicide attempts, patients with mood disorders have other emergencies, including psychotic breaks, anxiety attacks, extreme agitation, and homicidal or violent episodes.

The First 15 Minutes

As long as your patient is in a medical care unit, such as the psychiatry ward, there is minimal risk for the patient to harm himself or herself or others. However, the first 15 minutes of your evaluation of a depressed patient is going to set the tone for your relationship with your patient. Unless you suspect a medical issue underlying the patient's depressive episode, there is no reason to rush the psychiatric evaluation.

Initial Assessment

Skim through the patient's emergency room chart, including vital signs, and then quickly ensure that your patient is stable. If the patient appears unusually anxious, agitated, intoxicated, or disoriented, order an observer (sitter or security guard) at her side at all times as suicide risk is increased in these patient populations. If she is actively trying to harm herself, consider administering 1 to 2 mg Ativan by mouth or intramuscularly if she is unmanageable and refuses medications by mouth. If there is any concern that the patient has overdosed on medications, place a nasogastric tube, withdraw the stomach contents, and then administer activated charcoal through the nasogastric tube. Always check blood levels of the overdosed medication and then send for labs, including complete blood count (CBC) with differential, complete metabolic panel (CMP), other blood toxicology (e.g., for alcohol level), urine toxicology (e.g., illicit drugs), beta-HCG urine test (pregnancy test), urinalysis, and thyroid-stimulating hormone (TSH). Consider ordering rapid plasmin reagin (RPR) to rule out syphilis (not urgently—you may delay it at this point) and arterial blood gas (ABG) (if the patient appears ill, has respiratory symptoms, or reports overdosing).

Admission Criteria and Level of Care Criteria

Patients should be admitted to an inpatient psychiatric unit if they are medically stable and require 24-hour nursing or observation, are unable to care for themselves outside of the hospital, or it is anticipated that intensive medication changes will occur over a short period of time. Patients who lack capacity to sign a voluntary form or who are in imminent danger of hurting themselves or others should be involuntarily committed.

Patients who have overdosed on medications (especially aspirin, Tylenol, or tricyclic antidepressants) typically require admission to an intensive care unit (ICU) setting, followed by transfer to an inpatient psychiatry unit when medically stable. Stepping down to a medicine floor first is preferable but often not necessary. Patients who have cut their wrists should be evaluated and sutured as needed in the emergency room (ER). If the patient has been medically cleared by ER staff and a review of laboratory studies shows no gross abnormalities, proceed with an initial psychiatric history.

General guidelines for admitting a patient to an inpatient psychiatric bed versus discharging the patient to outpatient follow-up include the following:

1. Admit the patient if she is in imminent danger of harming herself or someone else. In other words, if she says she is suicidal, it is best to admit the patient unless you document clearly your rationale for discharge.
2. Admit the patient if she requires 24-hour nursing or supervision.
3. Admit the patient if it is anticipated that several medication trials or electroconvulsive therapy will be necessary.
4. Admit the patient if she is manic.
5. Admit the patient if her condition is affected to the degree that she cannot care for herself or children adequately.

Patients who are emergency petitioned are those who are brought to the ER at the request of other individuals who are concerned about the safety of the patient or others. In general, these patients should be admitted, unless you have spoken with the petitioner, the psychiatrist, and other key collateral people and you are confident she is safe for discharge. When you have decided to admit the patient to a psychiatric bed, she must sign a voluntary form that should be cosigned by a licensed physician. If the patient refuses to sign a voluntary form and you feel she requires inpatient admission, pursue involuntary hospitalization procedures. These procedures vary from state to state but typically require licensed physicians. Once a patient is transferred to the inpatient unit, she may decide she wants to leave because she is bored, isn't getting enough smoke breaks, or can't use drugs, for example. If this happens, have a voluntary patient sign a 72-hour notice (this may be handwritten on a progress note), which indicates her desire to be discharged. The patient may be held against her will for up to 72 hours from that time to give the primary team sufficient time to evaluate and begin treatment.

The First 24 Hours

The history is key to evaluating the psychiatric patient. Obtain what information you can in the ER and complete the initial workup on the floor.

History

Key elements of the history that you should obtain are the following:

• *Family history.* Obtain this information to assess genetic loading in the individual. Specifically ask about family members who have committed suicide or required inpatient psychiatric admission, as these are concrete parameters and indicate a greater severity of the mood disorders. Although the odds ratio of developing mood disorders in first-degree relatives is only about two compared to the general population, a family history of multiple members affected with severe mood disorder would lower your threshold for admission.

- *Personal history.* In psychiatric evaluations, knowing who the person is, where she came from, and what her expectations are in life are critical to understanding her current predicament. A more complete personal history may be obtained after admission to the floor, but try to get some basic information in the ER. If you are limited in time, ask the following three questions and move on: (i) *What did you parents do for a living?*, (ii) *What did people think of your parents when you were growing up?* (This question gets at the personalities of the parents.), and (iii) *What was your relationship like with your parents as a child?*

  On the floor, you want a more detailed history. Ask your patient where she was born and raised, what her home environment was like growing up; whether she was abused mentally, physically, or sexually, or was neglected (if she declines to answer, respect this and move on); what level of education she has achieved; her employment history (is she on disability?); her marital history; how many children she has; her living situation; and whether she is spiritual/religious. Obtain a brief legal history, including total jail time, violent arrests, and pending legal issues. Occasionally, patients attempt to avoid court dates by hiding out in hospitals, and patients who are under arrest legally should not be admitted to psychiatric units.

- *Substance abuse history.* Ask about cigarettes, alcohol, cocaine, heroin, marijuana, and other drugs of abuse, such as benzodiazepines (e.g., Valium, Klonopin, Xanax), opiates (e.g., OxyContin, Percocet, Tylox), LSD, and Ecstasy. Inquire about routes of administration. If the patient reports using intravenous drugs, consider offering HIV testing, and examine the patient for subcutaneous abscesses and auscultate the heart for murmurs indicative of endocarditis. Ask when she started using drugs, when she last used them, how much she uses, and history of withdrawal symptoms. Ask which detoxification or substance abuse programs she has enrolled in. Try to get a history for the patient's mood symptoms during periods of abstinence from drugs. This will be important in deciding whether the patient has a substance-induced mood disorder or a primary mood disorder.

- *Past psychiatric history.* Ask the patient who her current psychiatrist and/or therapist are, and get their phone numbers. Contact these individuals for collateral information in the ER if time allows or if the patient is not communicative. Otherwise, call them once the patient is admitted. Get information regarding the patient's premorbid (or baseline) personality and the onset of first mood symptoms. Get a description of a typical mood episode. Inquire about the number and location of psychiatric hospitalizations, suicide attempts (any in hospitals?), and other self-injurious behaviors (e.g., cutting). Get a history about any past medication trials. Screen for a history of manic episodes by asking, "Have you ever been sleepless for three nights straight? Did you have a lot of energy then?" If the patient answers yes and also reports pressured speech (people had difficulty interrupting her), flight of ideas (changing rapidly from topic to topic), grandiose ideas, increased libido, exorbitant spending, and a feeling of being "connected" with others, she likely had a manic episode. Less severe episodes that did not produce psychotic symptoms or impairment of function, or that result in hospitalization suggest hypomanic episodes. Psychosis is defined as being out of touch with reality and presents as hallucinations (perceptions without stimuli) and delusions (fixed, false, idiosyncratic beliefs). Screen for psychotic symptoms by asking whether the patient has ever had unusual experiences such as hearing voices or seeing things that are not there. Ask her if she has ever felt like she had supernatural powers or that individuals were conspiring against her. If she is adamant that it was true (it is fixed), but collateral informants prove it was false and the belief is not consistent with her upbringing, she is describing a history of a delusion.

• *History of the present illness.* Ask the patient what brought her to the hospital today. Look for triggering factors such as an argument with a significant other, recent homelessness, unemployment, poor work performance, or the death of a significant person. For patients reporting low mood and/or suicidal ideations, ask about depressive signs and symptoms using the mnemonic *SIGEMCAPS*:

• S = sleep (insomnia or hypersomnia)
• I = interest (anhedonia, lack of interest in having fun)
• G = guilt (low self attitude or self-worth)
• E = energy (typically decreased)
• M = mood (typically sad, but may be any dysphoric mood or dulling of mood)
• C = concentration (poor concentration or indecisiveness)
• A = appetite (decreased or, in atypical depression, increased)
• P = psychomotor (typically slowed with psychomotor retardation [PMR], but may have psychomotor agitation [PMA] in agitated depression)
• S = suicide (If the patient answers yes, ask about any plans. If the patient plans to use a gun and has access to one, take steps to remove this access.)

Physical Examination

The mental status examination (MSE) is the psychiatrist's version of the internist's physical examination and is critical for assessment and diagnosis. As a medical student, the most important part of your presentation to the attending is perhaps the MSE. Unlike the rest of the history, the MSE should be performed personally and not extracted from previous notes. For a complete outline of the MSE, see Chapter 1, Localization and the Neurologic Exam.

An example of an MSE for our depressed patient might read as follows:

The patient was a disheveled and malodorous Caucasian woman wearing a T-shirt and jeans. She was well-developed with no obvious physical abnormalities and appeared to be her stated age. She walked willingly to the examination room. Her gait was normal and her posture slouched. Significant psychomotor retardation was noted. There were no tremors or abnormal movements. She had poor eye contact with a frequent downcast look. Her speech was soft, slow, and monotonous, with notable response latency. Her thought processes were generally intact. She gave short, direct answers to questions. Her self-attitude was diminished in that she reported being ashamed of her productivity at work and envisioned little hope that she would ever be a respectable scholar. Her mood was self-described as "sad" and her affect was assessed as constricted and depressed. She denied hallucinations across all modalities. There were no delusions, panic attacks, obsessions, compulsions, or phobias. Her intelligence was at least average based on her vocabulary, abstraction abilities, general information, and educational achievement. She was alert and oriented and scored 27/30 on her Mini-Mental Status Exam (MMSE), missing two points for memory recall and one point for spelling "world" incorrectly.

Table 12-2 lists the mental status exam features that are common in depression and mania.

Labs and Tests to Consider

Although the patient has been medically cleared in the ER, you want to rule out common medical causes of depression. Make sure that the patient's TSH, RPR, and B12 levels are normal, as hypothyroidism, syphilis, and B12 deficiency are common medical causes of depression. Consider a CAT scan followed by MRI of the brain if the patient has new psychotic symptoms, focal neurologic signs, or an altered mental status. Left frontal brain infarcts traditionally produce depression, whereas anterior circulation injury results in abulia (lack of initiative) and a flat affect. Injuries to the right subcortical regions have been implicated in persistent mania. An electroencephalogram (EEG) should be considered in rare psychiatric presentations in which there is evidence of fluctuating consciousness or repetitive movements that suggest delirium or seizures, respectively.

Assessment

In addition to the MSE, attendings will focus on the formulation, which is essentially the assessment and plan for a psychiatric workup. The formulation should be about a paragraph long and should describe concisely key aspects of the patient's presentation, upbringing, personality, and past psychiatric history. A differential should be presented and discussed briefly, followed by initial plans and a prognosis. For our patient, a sample formulation might read as follows:

This is a 27-year-old Caucasian woman who grew up in a household with an alcoholic father and a mother who died at a young age during childbirth. Despite her chaotic upbringing, the patient has managed to pursue advanced studies in a

TABLE 12-2

Mental Status Exam Features Common to Depression and Mania

Exam	Features of Depression	Features of Mania
Appearance	Disheveled	Normal
Behavior	Slow in moving	Hyperactive
Speech	Slow in speaking	Rapid, difficult to interrupt
Affect	Appears sad	Euphoric
Thought process	Usually logical	May have elements of psychotic, bizarre thought process
Thought content	Usually reasonable but may ruminate; if illogical, think concurrent mania/psychosis	May have elements of psychotic, unusual thought content
Perceptions	Normal; if abnormal think medication effect	May have hallucinations, especially auditory
Cognition	Slow in thinking; poor concentration	Better than usual
Consciousness	May be reduced but should be easily arousable; if not, think drugs	Intact
Oriented	Normal	May believe he or she is a famous person
Memory	Poor working/short-term memory	Short-term memory impaired during manic period
Judgment	Normal	Poor
Insight	Good insight is a good prognostic factor	Good insight is a good prognostic factor

competitive program. Dimensionally, she is a stable introvert and these traits have served her well in her academic endeavors. She presents today with what appears to be her first episode of major depression. She reports no prior history of manias. There are no clear events that set off this depressive episode, and the picture is not complicated by illicit drugs per her toxicologies and self-reported history. Given the severity of her symptoms, including neurovegetative symptoms (psychomotor retardation, poor concentration, poor appetite) and a 2-week history of low mood and anhedonia, her case is formulated as a moderate, single episode of major depressive disorder. She will likely benefit from medication management together with psychotherapy. Inpatient psychiatric admission is recommended at this time because she reports ongoing suicidal ideation and does not appear able to care for herself or attend to her studies. Initiation of Wellbutrin or a selective serotonin reuptake inhibitor should be considered in this patient. She should attend occupational therapy groups for affective disorders. Given her unfamiliarity with the hospital setting and ongoing suicidal ideation, she will be placed on close observation overnight.

Treatment

Treatment for major depression begins on an inpatient basis on the psychiatry ward and continues in the outpatient psychiatry clinic on discharge. The inpatient care is focused on stabilizing the patient, ensuring to the best of your ability that the patient will not attempt suicide again and creating a comprehensive plan of antidepressant medication and psychotherapy.

Pharmacotherapy has evolved and expanded in the past 10 years. In the 1950s, tricyclic antidepressants including chlorpromazine and imipramine were the first widely used medications for mood disorders. With the relatively recent discovery of selective serotonin reuptake inhibitors (SSRIs), including fluoxetine (Prozac), therapy for depression usually involves a trial of SSRIs because of their superior safety and side-effect profiles. For patients with depression who suffer from psychomotor retardation, "activating" SSRIs that also block reuptake of norepinephrine and/or dopamine are alternative options. Table 12-3 lists the common medications used for mood disorders.

EXTENDED INHOSPITAL MANAGEMENT

The primary team should see the patient on rounds each morning and perform a tailored MSE, focusing on her subset of symptoms. In particular, ask about her self-attitude, mood, passive death wishes ("Is life worth living?") and suicidality (always ask about associated plans). It is also important to follow up on patients with mood disorders on vital senses, which includes her neurovegetative symptoms, such as fatigue as well as disturbances in sleep, appetite, and concentration. As psychotropics are added, be sure to ask about

TABLE 12-3
Pharmacotherapy for Mood Disorders

Indication	Drug Name	Adverse Effects
Depression	Fluoxetine (Prozac) Paroxetine (Paxil) Citalopram (Celexa) Escitalopram (Lexapro)	Drowsiness, dry mouth, nervousness, sexual dysfunction
	Venlafaxine (Effexor) Duloxetine (Cymbalta)	Same as above, plus withdrawal syndrome with discontinuation
	Mirtazapine (Remeron)	Increased appetite
	Bupropion (Wellbutrin)	Lowers seizure threshold
	Amitriptyline Imipramine	Anticholinergic symptoms (dry mouth, constipation, blurred vision). Toxic arrhythmias with overdose.
Depression (used to augment antidepressants above)	Risperidone (Risperdal) Olanzapine (Zyprexa) Quetiapine (Seroquel)	Tardive dyskinesias, blurred vision, muscle spasms, weight gain
Mania	Risperidone (Risperdal) Olanzapine (Zyprexa) Quetiapine (Seroquel)	Tardive dyskinesias, blurred vision, muscle spasms, weight gain
	Lithium	Thirst, tremors, light-headedness, nausea, diarrhea
	Carbamazepine (Tegretol) Lamotrigine (Lamictal)	Dizziness, drowsiness, nausea

side effects. It is better for the patient to report them without your having to list the side effects, as that may bias her answers. Side effects for Wellbutrin include seizures, especially in patients with alcoholism and bulimia. Anxiety and agitation are also relatively common side effects of Wellbutrin. Side effects for various SSRIs include headache, indigestion, nausea, and sexual side effects, such as decreased libido. The SSRIs with the most conservative side effect profiles are Celexa and Lexapro (Lexapro is similar to Celexa but has a better side-effect profile because only one enantiomer is present).

> **CLINICAL PEARL**
>
> *Be cautious using antidepressants in patients with histories of manias, as doing so may kindle and prolong the mania. Mania is treated acutely with an antipsychotic, and a mood stabilizer is required for maintenance. For this reason, it is important that you distinguish between depressive disorders and bipolar disorders. This is why we screen for mania in the past psychiatric history.*

DISPOSITION

Discharge Goals

There are several major discharge goals for patients with mood disorders:

• Improvement of mood back toward the baseline
• Improvement in affect and other symptoms of depression
• Denial of suicidal ideation
• Improvement in serial ratings on a depression scale. Examples include the Montgomery Asberg Depression Inventory or the Hamilton Depression Scale. A copy of the Hamilton Depression Scale is freely available on the internet at the Veterans Administration/Department of Defense Web site: http://www.oqp.med.va.gov/cpg/MDD/MDD_cpg/content/appendices/mdd_app1_fr.htm.

Outpatient Care

The patient should have outpatient follow-up arranged prior to discharge. If she is on psychotropic medications, she should see a psychiatrist for ongoing care and routine check of blood level check if on lithium or anticonvulsant medication. If she had presented with an adjustment disorder and did not require medication management, recommend follow-up with a therapist. Patients abusing substances should have substance abuse follow-up.

WHAT YOU NEED TO REMEMBER

- Mood disorders are diseases that produce episodic fluctuations in mood and include major depressive disorder, bipolar disorder type I, bipolar disorder type II, substance-induced mood disorders, and adjustment disorder.
- Up to 15% of depressed patients successfully commit suicide. Most of those patients attempt suicide by prescription medication overdose.
- The acute management of patients with mood disorders depends on the emergent situation. Substance overdose involves the administration of activated charcoal; anxiety, agitation, and psychosis may require psychoactive medications.
- A workup of mood disorders depends heavily on the history of the present illness, including the childhood history, social history, and family history.
- Long-term care for mood disorders includes both medication and psychotherapeutic strategies.

SUGGESTED READINGS

Cummings JL, Mega MS. *Neuropsychiatry and Behavioral Neuroscience.* Oxford, UK: Oxford University Press, 2003.

DePaulo JR Jr. *Understanding Depression.* New York: John Wiley and Sons, 2002.

Frances AJ, Ross R. *Diagnostic and Statistical Manual of Mental Disorders (DSM-IV-TR).* 4th Ed. text rev. Arlington, VA: American Psychiatric Association, 2003.

Kaufman DM. *Clinical Neurology for Psychiatrists.* Philadelphia: WB Saunders, 2006.

McHugh PR, Slavney PR. *The Perspectives of Psychiatry.* 2nd Ed. Baltimore: The Johns Hopkins University Press, 1998.

Tomb DA. *House Officer Series: Psychiatry.* 6th Ed. Philadelphia: Lippincott Williams & Wilkins, 1999.

CHAPTER

Schizophrenia

13

THE PATIENT ENCOUNTER

A 22-year-old man is emergency petitioned by his care provider who reports a 1-week history of talking to himself, insensible speech, and grossly disorganized and dangerous behaviors, including leaving a lit stove unattended and smearing feces on the sidewalk.

OVERVIEW

Definition and Pathophysiology

Schizophrenia is generally considered a chronic debilitating psychotic illness without return to baseline premorbid functioning. Emil Kraeplin originally named the illness dementia praecox (early-onset dementia) to differentiate it from mood disorders, which are typically episodic with full remission between exacerbations. Bleuler coined the term *schizophrenia* to describe the splitting of the cognitive processes, and went on to describe the four As of schizophrenia: (loose) associations, (inappropriate) affect, autistic withdrawal, and ambivalence. Schizophrenia is described in terms of positive symptoms (hallucinations, delusions) and negative symptoms (affective flattening, poverty of speech, avolition, anhedonia). Antipsychotics are more effective at treating the positive symptoms than they are the negative symptoms of schizophrenia.

The pathophysiology of schizophrenia has largely focused on the role of dopamine. Dopamine is a stimulatory neurotransmitter that, in excess, can cause psychosis. Blockers of the dopamine receptor, especially the D2-dopamine receptor, are effective in reducing the positive symptoms of schizophrenia, leading to the hypothesis that the pathophysiology of schizophrenia is a result of dopamine imbalance. But the role of dopamine does not account for all aspects of the disease. A newer antipsychotic, clozapine, improves the negative symptoms of schizophrenia through modulation of serotonergic receptors. Glutamatergic and nicotinic receptors are also being investigated as having a role in the pathogenesis of schizophrenia.

Recently, the first gene associated with the risk of schizophrenia has been identified. DARPP-32 (dopamine and cyclic AMP regulated phosphoprotein, 32 kilodalton) is involved in improved communication between the basal ganglia and the frontal lobe, where the protein is highly expressed. Some variants of DARPP-32 are thought to improve this communication but are also linked to an increased risk of schizophrenia. However, not all schizophrenic patients have this mutation and not all persons with this mutation will develop disease. More research is necessary to understand how DARPP-32 contributes to the pathogenesis of schizophrenia.

Patients with psychosis are out of touch with reality, and symptoms include hallucinations, delusions, disorganized speech, and grossly disorganized behavior. The differential for patients with psychotic symptoms is shown in Table 13-1.

TABLE 13-1
Differential Diagnoses of Psychosis

Diagnosis	Definition
Schizophrenia	Six months or more of psychosis with little mood component
Schizophreniform disorder	Psychotic symptoms 1–6 months in duration; many patients go on to develop schizophrenia
Schizoaffective disorder	Bipolar or depressed types; mood accounts for 1/3–2/3 of the entire time, and psychosis is present in absence of mood symptoms
Major depressive disorder with psychosis	Typical psychotic symptoms are mood congruent and limited to depressive episodes
Bipolar affective disorder, manic with psychosis	Psychotic symptoms typically mood congruent and limited to mood episodes
Substance-induced psychotic disorder	Symptoms are substance induced, for example, secondary to steroid or marijuana use
Delusional disorder	Hold nonbizarre delusions in the absence of any other symptoms of schizophrenia including hallucinations
Psychosis owing to a general medical condition	Symptoms are secondary, e.g., to hypercalcemia or celiac disease
Psychosis not otherwise specified	If symptoms do not fit above categories

Epidemiology

Schizophrenia affects roughly 1% of the population worldwide. Younger men who develop the illness have the worst prognosis and typically show signs in their early 20s. Women show signs in their late 20s, but schizophrenia can also emerge as late as age 45. There is a strong genetic predisposition; the risk of developing schizophrenia increases 9-fold if there is an affected sibling and 12-fold if there is an affected parent.

ACUTE MANAGEMENT AND WORKUP

Acute situations with schizophrenic patients most commonly involve controlling excessive positive symptoms, including psychosis and hallucinations. Negative symptoms such as cognitive problems and depression do not commonly lead to hospitalization and are managed on an outpatient basis.

The First 15 Minutes

Psychotic patients can be harmful to themselves, other patients, and the healthcare staff (including you!). Do not place yourself in harm's way and trust your gut instinct. The first 15 minutes are the most dangerous for you. Ask the medical guards to assist you in talking to and examining the patient. Remember: There is no shame in running away from a psychotic person.

Initial Assessment

Skim through the patient's emergency room chart, including vital signs, and then quickly ensure that your patient is stable. If the patient appears unusually anxious, agitated, intoxicated, or disoriented, order an observer at his side at all times to prevent dangerous behaviors. If he is actively thrashing about and there is concern for physical harm to the patient or others, order a cocktail of lorazepam (Ativan) 1 to 2 mg, haloperidol (Haldol) 5 mg, and diphenhydramine (Benadryl) 25 to 50 mg. Offer to administer by mouth (PO), but if he refuses, administer via intramuscular (IM) injection. Intravenous (IV) administration is also acceptable, but most psychiatric patients will not have a Hep-Lock IV available. If, after 10 minutes, the patient continues with physically violent maneuvers, administer a second round of the above cocktail.

Remember that Ativan is a benzodiazepine and therefore produces respiratory depression in overdose. Keep track of how much Ativan you are ordering. Use caution in patients with respiratory disorders, and, as a general rule, do not give more than 6 mg in a day unless the patient is in alcohol or benzodiazepine withdrawal. Haloperidol is an antipsychotic that may produce an acute dystonic reaction, such as oculogyric crisis (eyes rolling up) or torticollis (neck flexion), which are extremely uncomfortable. Diphenhydramine 50 mg (PO/IM) or benztropine (Cogentin) 1 mg (PO/IM) should be administered if the patient develops a dystonic reaction. Haldol can also prolong the QT interval and is contraindicated in cases of known heart disease. If the patient is this agitated, he will also require placement in locked-door or open-door seclusion, where he will be monitored via video and separated from other patients. Restraints are reserved for desperate cases in which the patient's actions continue to present an immediate danger to himself or others.

Conversely, many schizophrenic patients with acute psychoses are very guarded, quiet, and may even be catatonic. If the patient is not communicative, it is best to get a constant observer. If he appears to be responding to internal stimuli such as voices, consider offering oral medications, including an atypical antipsychotic such as risperidol (Risperdal) 4 mg or olanzapine (Zyprexa) 5 mg. Lorazepam (Ativan) 1 mg may be offered for catatonic symptoms (waxy flexibility, mutism, immobility) or anxiety.

CLINICAL PEARL

Newer atypical antipsychotic drugs now come in an optional rapidly dissolving form that prevents patients from "cheeking" their pills and spitting them out later.

Send for basic labs, including complete blood count (CBC) with differential, complete metabolic panel (CMP), blood toxicology (for alcohol level), urine toxicology, urinalysis, and thyroid-stimulating hormone (TSH).

Admission Criteria and Level of Care Criteria

General guidelines for admitting psychotic patients to an inpatient psychiatric bed versus discharging to outpatient follow-up include the following considerations. Admit the patient if:

- He is in imminent danger of harming himself or someone else, whether this is intentional or not.
- He requires 24-hour nursing or supervision.
- It is anticipated that several medication trials or electroconvulsive therapy will be necessary.
- His condition is affected to the degree that he cannot care for himself or dependents adequately.
- This is a first psychotic episode ("psychotic break").

Patients who are emergency petitioned are those who are brought to the ER at the request of other individuals who are concerned about the safety of the patient or his effects on others. In general, these patients should be admitted, unless you have spoken with the petitioner, the psychiatrist, and other key collateral people and you are confident he is safe for discharge.

There are two main types of admission: voluntary and involuntary. If a psychotic patient demonstrates comprehension of the voluntary admission form and agrees to sign it, he should be admitted voluntarily. If he lacks capacity to understand the form or refuses to sign it and your judgment is that he needs to be hospitalized, activate involuntary admission procedures.

The First 24 Hours

As with patients with mood disorders, a good psychiatric history is key. However, psychotic patients are often unable to provide this information. Therefore, it is important to use collateral informants and previous records.

History

Key elements of the history that you should obtain are the following:

- *Family history.* Obtain this information to assess genetic loading in the individual. The monozygotic concordance of schizophrenia is roughly 50%, suggesting both genetic and environmental causes for the disorder. Rates of mood disorders are typically elevated in family members of patients with schizophrenia, so ask about the family history of psychiatric illness in general. Specifically ask about family members who have committed suicide or required inpatient psychiatric admission, as these are concrete parameters and indicate a greater severity of disease.

> **CLINICAL PEARL**
>
> *Thirty percent of patients with schizophrenia attempt suicide, and 10% complete it.*

- *Personal history.* In psychiatric evaluations, knowing who the patient is and what his formidable experiences are in life are critical to understanding his current predicament. This also pertains to patients with schizophrenia, who are likely to appear more disengaged than they feel. A more complete personal history may be obtained after admission to the floor, but try to get some basic information in the ER. If you are limited in time, ask the following three questions: (i) *What did your parents do for a living?*, (ii) *What did people think of your parents when you were growing up?*, (This question gets at the personalities of the parents.), and (iii) *What was your relationship like with your parents as a child?*

  On the floor, you want a more detailed history. Ask your patient where he was born and raised; what his home environment was like growing up; whether he was abused physically, emotionally, or sexually, or was neglected (if he declines to answer, respect this and move on); what level of education he has achieved; his employment history (is he on disability?);

his marital history; how many children he has; his living situation; and whether he is spiritual/religious. Obtain a brief legal history, including total jail time, violent arrests, and pending legal issues. Occasionally, patients attempt to avoid court dates by hiding out in hospitals, and patients who are under arrest legally should not be admitted to psychiatric units.

- *Substance abuse history.* It is estimated that among patients with schizophrenia, more than 80% smoke cigarettes and about 50% abuse another substance. A substantial portion of patients with schizophrenia report a heavy period of marijuana use prior to the first psychotic break. Conversely, there are cases in which patients develop acute psychosis in the setting of substance abuse (especially marijuana), but the psychotic episode resolves spontaneously. For these reasons, it is important to ascertain the timeline for substance abuse and psychotic symptoms.

  In establishing the patient's substance abuse history, ask about cigarettes, alcohol, cocaine, heroin, marijuana, and other drugs of abuse, such as benzodiazepines (e.g., Valium, Klonopin, Xanax), opiates (e.g., OxyContin, Percocet, Tylox), LSD, and Ecstasy. Inquire about routes of administration. If the patient reports using intravenous drugs, consider offering HIV testing, and examine the patient for subcutaneous abscesses and auscultate the heart for murmurs indicative of endocarditis. Ask when he last used various drugs. Ask which detoxification or substance abuse programs he has enrolled in. Get a history of the patient's psychotic symptoms during periods of abstinence from drugs. This will aid you in determining whether the patient has a substance-induced psychotic disorder or schizophrenia.

- *Past psychiatric history.* Ask the patient who his current psychiatrist and/or therapist are, and get their phone numbers. Contact these individuals for collateral information in the ER if time allows or if the patient is not communicative. Otherwise, call them once the patient is admitted. Ask the patient to describe when he first experienced psychotic symptoms and how they manifested.

  Remember, psychosis is defined as being out of touch with reality. Psychosis is manifested as hallucinations (perceptions without stimuli) and delusions (fixed, false, idiosyncratic beliefs). Auditory hallucinations are the most common kind of hallucinations in schizophrenia. If a patient reports visual hallucinations, consider delirium related to benzodiazepine or alcohol withdrawal or an organic brain process, such as a brain tumor. If a patient reports olfactory hallucinations, consider a seizure disorder. It is also important to distinguish between a hallucination and an illusion, which is a misinterpretation of a real stimulus. Examples of illusions include seeing potted plants as purring cats, or hearing a pounding hammer as an intruder stomping down the hallway.

  There are also what are called pseudohallucinations, which are essentially vaguely described hallucinations. Examples of pseudohallucinations are shadows moving in the peripheral vision (as opposed to clearly delineated objects) or voices that are difficult to pinpoint in location and in the content of what they say although they often reflect the patient's own thoughts. Pseudohallucinations may clarify into hallucinations with the progression of illness; therefore, they should not be taken lightly. Still, clear-cut hallucinations provide stronger evidence for schizophrenia. Try to get as much detail on the hallucinations as possible, as the content and forms of hallucinations may help differentiate psychosis secondary to schizophrenia versus a mood disorder. As a general rule, patients with mood disorders have hallucinations that are mood congruent (e.g., hearing derogatory comments while in a depressed state). However, patients with schizophrenia have hallucinations constantly regardless of mood state, and the hallucinations may be mood incongruent and/or bizarre (e.g., hearing voices talking about aliens living in the television while in a euthymic state). The forms of the hallucinations are also helpful in differentiating psychosis secondary to a mood state versus schizophrenia. Patients with textbook schizophrenia typically hear more than two voices in great detail, can point to where the voices are coming from, and describe the voices arguing with each other or commenting on the patient's actions in the third person.

Last, get a history of mood symptoms (see Chapter 12, Mood Disorders) and how they relate to psychotic symptoms. Although the incidence of comorbid mood disorders is high in schizophrenia, what you are trying to identify is whether the mood disorder is *always* present with the psychosis. If the patient has had psychotic symptoms continuously for more than 6 months with a relative *absence* of mood symptoms, he likely has schizophrenia. If the patient has psychotic symptoms *only and always* related to alterations in mood states, he likely has major depressive disorder with psychotic symptoms or bipolar affective disorder, manic with psychosis. If he has prominent mood symptoms for one third to two thirds of the time and with ongoing psychotic symptoms in the absence of mood disturbance, he may receive a diagnosis of schizoaffective disorder.

- *History of the present illness.* Ask the patient what brought him to the hospital today. If you are unable to obtain an answer, ask collateral informants.

Physical Examination

The mental status exam (MSE) is the psychiatrist's version of the internist's physical examination and is critical for assessment and diagnosis. As a medical student, the most important part of your presentation to the attending is perhaps the MSE. Unlike the rest of the history, the MSE should be performed personally and not extracted from previous notes. For a complete outline of the MSE, see Chapter 1, Localization and the Neurologic Exam.

An example of an MSE for our psychotic patient might read as follows:

The patient was a disheveled, thin Caucasian man with long hair and a beard who was wearing a hospital gown. He sat vigilantly in a chair to one side of the open door of the seclusion room. He made few movements, but when he did, he was not noted to be psychomotor agitated nor retarded. He was guarded but allowed a brief examination. There was no waxy flexibility. His speech was soft, slow, and monotonous. There was evidence of formal thought disorder in the form of loosening of associations. He spoke in long sentences with an impressive vocabulary, but his sentences often did not relate to one another. He described his mood as "fine" and he appeared suspicious with a blunted affect. His self-attitude was fair in that he felt he was a good person who had things to offer this world, but he expressed some skepticism about the future. He stated that his sleep, energy, concentration, and appetite have been "fine," indicating preserved vital sense. However he seemed inattentive at times (poor concentration) and he was very thin, indicating poor intake by mouth. He denied passive death wishes and suicidal ideation, but described homicidal ideation in the form of a voice that kept telling him to stab his roommate (command hallucination). He had auditory hallucinations, which he described as several men and women arguing with each other. He did not recognize these voices as people he knows. They were outside of his head and originated from a location several feet from his right ear. Sometimes, one of the male voices would comment on his actions continuously in the third person. The voices made positive, negative, and neutral comments that did not necessarily correlate with the patient's mood. He denied hallucinations in other modalities. He had the delusion that these voices were spirits of his great-grandchildren, who would be born as robots. He also had passivity signs, including that these spirits could control his bodily movements and emotions. There were no obsessions, compulsions, anxiety, panic attacks, and phobias. His intelligence was considered to be average based on his vocabulary and educational achievement, but with his illness, he has likely lost significant cognitive points. He had poor abstraction abilities. His Mini-Mental State Examination was 25/30; he missed two points for orientation, two points for serial sevens, and one point for failing to follow a complex command.

Table 13-2 lists the mental status exam features that are common in schizophrenia.

Labs and Tests to Consider

Although the patient has been medically cleared in the ER, you want to rule out common medical causes of psychiatric disease. It is standard to check levels of TSH, B12, and rapid plasmin reagin (RPR). For patients presenting with their first episode of psychotic symptoms, order a CAT scan followed by MRI of the brain along with an encephalogram (EEG). Rarely, tumors, strokes, or seizures may be the cause of psychotic

TABLE 13-2
Mental Status Exam Features Common to Schizophrenia

Mental Status Exam	Features
Appearance	Disheveled
Behavior	Ambivalent to take any actions
Speech	Often incoherent
Affect	Blunted, flat, or inappropriate
Thought process	Bizarre, idiosyncratic thinking
Thought content	Preoccupation with vague philosophic ideas; delusions
Perceptions	Hallucinations
Cognition	Intact but difficult to assess
Consciousness	Intact but emotionally distant from interviewer
Oriented	Confused about identity; confused about the meaning of life
Memory	Poor working/short-term memory
Judgment	Poor
Insight	Usually poor

symptoms, and in such cases, you would not want to give a life-altering diagnosis of schizophrenia. Beware of anterior circulation infarcts that typically produce abulia, which resembles the catatonic state. Other causes of psychosis include steroid use, celiac disease, systemic lupus erythematosus, porphyria, pellagra, Parkinson's dementia, Lewy body dementia, Alzheimer's dementia, Huntington's disease, Sydenham chorea, Wilson disease, hypercalcemia, hyponatremia, uremia, hepatic encephalopathy, and heavy metal intoxication.

Assessment

In addition to the MSE, attendings will focus on the formulation, which is essentially the assessment and plan for a psychiatric workup. The formulation should be about a paragraph long and should describe concisely key aspects of the patient's presentation, upbringing, personality, and past psychiatric history. A differential should be presented and discussed briefly, followed by initial plans and prognosis. For our patient, a sample formulation might read as follows:

This is a 22-year-old single Caucasian man with a prior diagnosis of schizophrenia and multiple past admissions for exacerbations of his illness. He was emergency petitioned after he left on a lit gas stove and was found smearing feces along a sidewalk. According to prior records, he was raised in a financially middle class home by a father who was an accountant and a mother who was a homemaker. The patient was an only child, and he had few friends growing up. Premorbidly, he was quiet and was described by his mother as a difficult child prone to irritable outbursts (unstable introvert). He was an average student until his sophomore year in college, when he severely withdrew and failed all of his classes. He was found in his dorm room not having eaten or bathed in days and was noted to be self-dialoguing. He was admitted to the University Hospital, where he underwent electroconvulsive therapy as well as trials of Haldol, lithium, and Prolixin. His case was initially formulated with the diagnosis of bipolar disorder, but in subsequent years it was reformulated with schizophrenia. Over the past 8 years, he has been admitted to psychiatric inpatient units more than eight times and he has been tried on multiple antipsychotics, including intramuscular depot injections. His course has been chronic and progressive without return to baseline, supporting a diagnosis of schizophrenia. Over the past 3 years, he has done reasonably well in a group home setting but continues to require inpatient admission every couple of years. Given his current condition, inpatient admission is warranted and he will require constant observation given his severely disorganized state and command hallucinations to harm an individual. In reviewing prior records, he has not been tried on Clozaril and his WBC [white blood count] and ANC [absolute neutrophil count] are within normal ranges; therefore, we will begin treatment with Clozaril.

Treatment

The mainstay of treatment of schizophrenia is antipsychotics, including traditional neuroleptics (Haldol, Prolixin) as well as atypical antipsychotics (Risperdal, Invega, Zyprexa, Geodon, Seroquel, Abilify, Clozaril), which produce fewer dystonic reactions. Patients with advanced illness and noncompliance typically require intramuscular depots given every 2 to 4 weeks. Patients should be monitored for cogwheeling rigidity regularly to assess for Parkinsonism and dystonic reactions secondary to antipsychotics. Cogentin is often prescribed to prevent dystonic reactions. Clozaril should be prescribed as a last resort if other medications fail to produce results. Clozaril is the only antipsychotic that has been shown to decrease suicide in patients with schizophrenia and is highly efficacious. However, there is a rare risk of developing agranulocytosis and, consequently, a weekly CBC is required early in treatment. Table 13-3 summarizes the common antipsychotics used to treat schizophrenia.

TABLE 13-3
Pharmacotherapy for Psychotic Disorders

Drug Name	Short or Long Acting	When to Use	Adverse Effects
Haloperidol (Haldol)	Short	Indication: acute psychosis Contraindication: known heart disease	Tardive dyskinesia, akathisia, dry mouth, lethargy, neuroleptic malignant syndrome
Fluphenazine (Prolixin)	Short	Indication: acute psychosis	Tardive dyskinesia, akathisia, dry mouth, lethargy, neuroleptic malignant syndrome
Risperidone (Risperdal), Olanzapine (Zyprexa) Quetiapine (Seroquel)	Long	Indication: first line therapy for schizophrenia and psychotic disorders	Less incidence of tardive dyskinesia compared to haloperidol; watch for hyperglycemia, weight gain, and diabetes
Clozapine (Clozaril)	Long	Indication: treatment-resistant schizophrenia	Agranulocytosis

Finally, involvement of the family and teaching social support skills is critical to improving the quality of life for patients with schizophrenia. Remember, part of the illness involves a disconnect between feeling (inside) and affect (expression on the face or body language). It is important to make a real effort to make the patient feel comfortable with you. It is also important for you not to feel discouraged if he appears disinterested or overly reserved. With constant warm support, most patients will start to open up to you.

EXTENDED INHOSPITAL MANAGEMENT

The primary team should see the patient on rounds each morning and perform a tailored MSE, focusing on his subset of symptoms. For patients with schizophrenia, ask about mood, passive death wishes, suicidal and homicidal ideation, paranoia, hallucinations, delusions, passivity signs, and anxiety. Use a genuine and direct approach. Do not try to be overly sweet or humorous, as these approaches may make it difficult for the patient to trust you.

DISPOSITION

Discharge Goals

The primary discharge goal for patients with schizophrenia is improvement of psychotic symptoms back to baseline or to a degree that the patient does not require 24-hour supervision. Many patients with schizophrenia will continue to have residual psychotic symptoms, even on medications. As long as the patient is not overly paranoid or anxious, and is reasonably organized enough to keep out of danger and does not require constant observation or nursing, he is safe for discharge. Depending on the severity of symptoms, he may be appropriate for discharge to a day hospital, day program, group home, or his own home (if he is higher functioning).

Outpatient Care

The patient should have outpatient follow-up arranged prior to discharge, and this information should be relayed in writing to his care provider at his group home. Given the rare but serious complication of agranulocytosis with Clozaril, the patient will need weekly CBC and ANC measurements for the first 6 months of treatment. This should be made explicit in the discharge instructions.

WHAT YOU NEED TO REMEMBER

- Schizophrenia is generally considered a chronic debilitating psychotic illness without return to baseline premorbid functioning.
- Schizophrenia is described in terms of positive symptoms (hallucinations, delusions) and negative symptoms (affective flattening, poverty of speech, avolition, anhedonia).
- Acute management of an actively psychotic patient who is a danger to himself or others includes being treated with a cocktail of lorazepam (Ativan) 1 to 2 mg, haloperidol (Haldol) 5 mg, and diphenhydramine (Benadryl) 25 to 50 mg.
- A good history is important to understand the exact nature of the psychosis and will guide therapy.
- Treatment is focused on administering antipsychotic medications plus treating comorbid conditions, such as mood disorders.

SUGGESTED READINGS

Andreasen NC, Black DW. *Introductory Textbook of Psychiatry*. Arlington, VA: American Psychiatry Publishing, 2001.

Cummings JL, Mega MS. *Neuropsychiatry and Behavioral Neuroscience*. Oxford, UK: Oxford University Press, 2003.

Frances AJ, Ross R. *Diagnostic and Statistical Manual of Mental Disorders (DSM-IV-TR)*. 4th Ed text rev. Arlington, VA: American Psychiatric Association, 2003.

Kaufman DM. *Clinical Neurology for Psychiatrists*. Philadelphia: WB Saunders, 2006.

McHugh PR, Slavney PR. *The Perspectives of Psychiatry*. 2nd Ed. Baltimore: The Johns Hopkins University Press, 1998.

Tomb DA. *House Officer Series: Psychiatry*. 6th Ed. Philadelphia: Lippincott Williams & Wilkins, 1999.

14

Personality Disorders

A 31-year-old single woman is brought to the emergency room via ambulance after she called 911 and self-reported a suicide attempt of cutting her forearms and wrists.

OVERVIEW

Definition and Pathophysiology

Personality disorders are pervasive disorders of character styles that produce impairment in relationships and career. In general, patients with personality disorders typically have poor insight into them, and medications and short-term therapy are ineffective at reversing symptoms. Personality disorders are differentiated from mood disorders, the latter of which have a waxing and waning episodic nature with the mood disturbances. Individuals with personality disorders may experience worsening of symptoms during periods of stress, but they have the signs and symptoms of the disorder at all times. Personality disorders, along with mental retardation, are coded on axis II of the DSM, unlike other psychiatric diseases, such as mood disorders, schizophrenia, and substance abuse, which are coded on axis I.

Think of axis II disorders as dimensional disorders. In other words, these types of disorders (i.e., of personality and intelligence) come in ranges. They are not categorical like schizophrenia or bipolar disorder, which an individual either has or does not have. An individual can be very intelligent, of average intelligence, or not so intelligent. Likewise, people may be quiet, outgoing, planners, able to work in the moment, timid, or aggressive. In moderation, these traits are not problematic and, in fact, may be beneficial. However, if the traits become too rigid and severe, the patient may have pervasive problems in interpersonal relations and in his or her career, and may receive a diagnosis of a personality disorder.

There are three main clusters of personality disorders:

A: Odd and eccentric. Includes paranoid, schizoid, and schizotypal personality disorders
B: Dramatic. Includes histrionic, narcissistic, borderline personality, and antisocial personality disorders

C: Anxious. Includes avoidant, dependent, and obsessive-compulsive personality disorders

A full description of all of the personality disorders would encompass an entire book in and of itself. Table 14-1 lists the key points about each personality disorder to aid in your diagnosis of a patient with a lifelong pattern of problems secondary to severe personality traits.

Longitudinal studies of physical and sexual abuse in childhood have consistently been linked to personality disorders of all types in adults. Physical abuse is particularly associated with antisocial personality disorder.

Epidemiology

According to the only national study of personality disorders that surveyed 43,093 American adults, 14.79% of us have at least one personality disorder (1). In order, the most common personality disorders are as follows:

1. Obsessive-compulsive (7.88%)
2. Paranoid (4.41%)
3. Antisocial (3.63%)
4. Schizoid (3.13%)
5. Avoidant (2.36%)
6. Histrionic (1.84%)
7. Dependent (0.49%)

Borderline, schizotypal, and narcissistic personality disorders were not assessed in this study but would have certainly pushed the fraction of affected Americans to more than 15%. It was difficult to tease out a difference between the prevalence of personality disorders in men and women, but in general, antisocial personality disorders are more common in men and dependent personality disorders are more common in women.

ACUTE MANAGEMENT AND WORKUP

Patients with personality disorders are often described as difficult, manipulative, and evoking a strong, negative countertransference (i.e., you don't like her). It's okay to keep in mind that a patient likely has a personality disorder, but try to hold final judgment until you have ruled out other psychiatric disease. It would not serve the patient well to receive a diagnosis of borderline personality disorder if she is really manifesting a mixed manic state, an agitated depressed state, or the effect of a substance.

The First 15 Minutes

In the first 15 minutes of managing patients with personality disorders, consider spending most of that time preparing yourself for the difficulty of dealing with these disorders.

TABLE 14-1

Clusters of Personality Disorders

Personality Disorder		DSM-IV Descriptors
A	Paranoid	Distrust and suspiciousness of others that their motives are malevolent or exploitive. Preoccupied with loyalty and trustworthiness
	Schizoid	Detached from social relationships, restricted range of expression of emotions, solitary, indifferent to praise and criticism, enjoys few activities
	Schizotypal	Reduced capacity for close relationships, eccentric beliefs and behaviors, odd and vague speech, bizarre fantasies
B	Histrionic	Excessive emotionality and attention-seeking, uncomfortable not being the center of attention, sexually seductive or provocative, impressionistic speech lacking in detail
	Narcissistic	Grandiosity, exaggerates achievements and talents, need for admiration, sense of entitlement, lack of empathy, exploitive of others, arrogant and haughty actions, 'empty' feelings, only thinks of self. Often based on sense of insecurity
	Borderline	Unstable and intense relationships, impulsive, fear of abandonment with frantic efforts to avoid it, recurrent suicidal or self-mutilating behaviors, chronic feelings of emptiness, difficulty controlling anger
	Antisocial	Disregard for and violation of the rights of others, repeated arrests, failure to conform with social norms, deceitfulness, lying, impulsive and aggressive resulting in repeated fights, irritable, irresponsible with work or financial obligations

TABLE 14-1

Clusters of Personality Disorders (Continued)

Personality Disorder		DSM-IV Descriptors
C	Avoidant	Social inhibition, feelings of inadequacy, hypersensitivity to rejection, avoids occupational situations for fear of criticism, unwilling to get involved with people unless certain of being liked
	Dependent	Need to be taken care of, submissive, clinging, fear of separation, difficulty making everyday decisions without reassurance, difficulty expressing disagreement for fear of loss of support/approval, needs others to assume responsibility, uncomfortable being alone
	Obsessive-compulsive	Orderliness, perfectionism, demands mental and physical control (inflexible), preoccupied with rules and lists, excessively devoted to work at the expense of friendships and leisure activities, reluctant to delegate tasks to others unless things are done exactly his or her way, miserly, overconscientious

Initial Assessment

Skim through the patient's emergency room chart, including vital signs, and then quickly ensure that your patient is stable. Look at her arm wounds and determine whether they require suturing. This is typically done by the emergency room resident prior to obtaining a psychiatric consult. Note the patient's general mental state. If she appears unusually anxious, agitated, intoxicated, or disoriented, or has just attempted suicide, as in the case study patient, order an observer at her side at all times.

Medicate the patient if she is actively thrashing about and there is concern for physical harm to herself or others. Start with Ativan 1 to 2 mg by mouth. If this fails to calm her and she is physically out of control, administer the standard cocktail for severely agitated patients: Ativan (1–2 mg), Haldol (5 mg) and Benadryl (25–50 mg). Offer to administer these by mouth (PO), but if she refuses, administer them via intramuscular (IM) injection.

Intravenous (IV) administration is also acceptable, but most psychiatric patients will not have a Hep-Lock IV available.

Send for labs, including complete blood count (CBC) with differential, complete metabolic panel (CMP), blood toxicology (for alcohol level), urine toxicology, urinalysis, and thyroid-stimulating hormone (TSH).

Admission Criteria and Level of Care Criteria

General guidelines for admitting patients to an inpatient psychiatric bed versus discharging to outpatient follow-up include the following considerations. Admit the patient under the following circumstances:

- She is in imminent danger of harming herself or someone else. In other words, if she reports ongoing suicidal ideations, it is best to admit unless you clearly have a rationale for discharge.
- She requires 24-hour nursing or supervision.
- It is anticipated that several medication trials or electroconvulsive therapy will be necessary
- Her condition is affected to the degree that she cannot care for herself or dependents adequately

CLINICAL PEARL

Personality disorders are not billable for inpatient admissions. You will therefore rarely (if ever) see an inpatient discharge summary with only a personality disorder (listed on axis II). There will typically be a coexisting mood disorder or other psychiatric diagnosis listed on axis I. This is not to say that patients with personality disorders don't require inpatient admissions. In deciding whether or not to admit, use the guidelines noted previously, together with your clinical skills.

There are two main types of admission: voluntary and involuntary. If the patient would benefit from admission and comprehends the voluntary form and agrees to sign it, admit her as a voluntary admission. If she lacks the capacity to understand the form or refuses to sign it and your judgment is that she needs to be hospitalized, activate involuntary admission procedures.

The First 24 Hours

A good psychiatric history is key to proper diagnosis and treatment. Get as much information as you can in the emergency room and complete the history on the floor. Use collateral informants and old records as psychiatric patients in the midst of illness are often unable to provide a complete history.

History

Key elements of the history that you should obtain are the following:

- *Family history.* Obtain this information to assess genetic loading in the individual. Specifically ask about family members who have committed suicide or required inpatient psychiatric admission as these are concrete parameters and indicate a greater severity of disease.
- *Personal history.* In psychiatric evaluations, knowing who the patient is and what her formidable experiences are in life are critical to understanding her current predicament. If you are limited in time, ask the following three questions: (i) *What did your parents do for a living?* (ii) *What did people think of your parents when you were growing up?* (This question gets at the personalities of the parents.), and (iii) *What was your relationship like with your parents as a child?* On the floor, you want a more detailed history. Ask your patient where she was born and raised; what her home environment was like growing up; whether she was abused physically, emotionally, or sexually, or was neglected (if she declines to answer, respect this and move on); what level of education she has achieved; her employment history (is she on disability?); her marital history; how many children she has; her living situation; and whether she is spiritual/religious. Obtain a brief legal history, including total jail time, violent arrests, and pending legal issues. Occasionally, patients attempt to avoid court dates by hiding out in hospitals, and patients who are under arrest legally should not be admitted to psychiatric units. For patients with borderline personality disorder, ask in particular about abuse history. Also inquire about early relationships that were unpredictable, such as a mother who was prone to highly variable mood states.
- *Substance abuse history.* For every substance, ask the patient how much and how often she uses, her first use, her most recent use, the route of administration, and whether she has had withdrawal signs or symptoms. In establishing the patient's substance abuse history, ask about alcohol, cigarettes, heroin, cocaine, marijuana, and other drugs of abuse, such as benzodiazepines (Ativan, Xanax, Klonopin, Valium), narcotics (Percocet, Tylox, Dilaudid, Vicodin), hallucinogens (Ecstasy, LSD), inhalants (paint thinner), as well as any other drugs she uses. Ask about any history of detoxification and substance abuse programs and whether these were helpful. As with all psychiatric illnesses, get an idea of her symptoms when she is abstinent from drugs to ascertain whether her symptoms are secondary to drug use versus a primary illness.
- *Past psychiatric history.* Ask the patient who her current psychiatrist and/or therapist are, and get their phone numbers. Contact these individuals for collateral information in the ER if time allows or once the patient is admitted. Get a premorbid personality profile from the patient and a reliable outside informant. To screen for a history of

depression, ask about sustained periods of low mood, feelings of guilt/self-deprecation, and neurovegetative symptoms. To qualify for a major depressive episode, the episode has to last for 2 weeks or longer. To screen for a history of manias, ask about periods during which she did not sleep for 3 days or more and had high energy and high mood. To qualify for a manic episode, she must report abstinence from drugs (especially cocaine) at the time and the duration of symptoms should be at least 1 week. If the patient describes reactive mood states that are situationally motivated and fluctuate multiple times during the day, strongly consider an underlying personality disorder. Finally, screen for a history of psychotic symptoms by asking about hallucinations and delusions, and also ask about anxiety, panic attacks, obsessions, compulsions, and phobias.

• *History of the present illness.* Ask the patient what brought her to the hospital today. Look for triggering factors, such as an argument with a significant other, a job loss, or a relapse into substance use. If there is no clear evidence of a mood episode or psychotic symptoms, she may be acting out to gain sympathy. This is characteristic of patients with borderline personality disorder (BPD). Thus, if you suspect your patient has BPD, give her the attention she is seeking and listen to her story. She may relay that she had no intention of dying, but was desperate to connect with someone. Try to empathize with her, but remember to keep firm boundaries with BPD patients. Maintain your professionalism and do not give her the impression that she is getting special treatment.

Physical Examination

The MSE is the psychiatrist's version of the internist's physical examination and is critical for assessment and diagnosis. As a medical student, the most important part of your presentation to the attending is perhaps the MSE. Unlike the rest of the history, the MSE should be performed personally and not extracted from previous notes. For a complete outline of the MSE, see Chapter 1, Localization and the Neurologic Exam.

Among the personality disorders, borderline personality disorder is one that you will likely encounter in the inpatient setting. An example of an MSE for our patient with borderline personality disorder might read as follows:

The patient was an overweight woman with fair skin and dyed black hair who appeared to be her stated age. She had numerous piercings in her ears, nose, tongue, and eyebrows. She sat in her bed as she glared with a piercing stare. Her anterior forearms revealed more than 50 superficial cuts consistent with her history of self-inflicted cutting with razors. There were wounds in various stages of healing, and there were more cuts on the left arm (she is right-handed). They were oriented perpendicular to the length of her arms. There were seven fresh cuts on her right forearm; none was deep enough to require sutures. There was no evidence of infection from the wounds. There were no abnormal movements. There was no psychomotor agitation or retardation. Her speech was regular in rate, rhythm, volume, and tone, and was goal oriented. She made frequent sarcastic comments, which served to denigrate ER staff and idealize her outpatient therapist. Her mood was self-described as "empty . . . angry" and her mood was assessed as irritable and dysphoric. Her affect was mood congruent and full range. Her self-attitude was low in that she described herself as a "pathetic person." She described vital senses (concentration, sleep, energy, appetite) that were largely intact. Hallucinations were absent in all modalities. There were no delusions, anxiety, obsessions, compulsions, and phobias (N.B.: Her self-cutting is not an obsession or compulsion because it is egosyntonic, meaning that the self-cutting makes her feel good rather than anxious). Her intelligence was considered to be at least average based on her language, abstraction abilities, and educational achievement. Her Mini-Mental State Exam was 30/30.

Table 14-2 lists the mental status exam features that are common in borderline personality disorder.

Labs and Tests to Consider

Although the patient has been medically cleared in the ER, you want to rule out common medical causes of psychiatric disease. It is standard to check levels of thyroid-stimulating hormone (TSH), B12, and rapid plasmin reagin (RPR). In patients who have a sudden change of personality, particularly if there is concomitant history of head trauma or if the patient is elderly, consider brain imaging studies. Personality changes are associated with frontal tumors, such as slow-growing meningiomas, which have been known to grow to significant sizes before focal neurologic exams are observed.

Assessment

In addition to the MSE, attendings will focus on your formulation, which is essentially the assessment and plan for a psychiatric workup. The formulation should be about a paragraph long and should describe concisely key aspects of the patient's presentation, upbringing, personality, and past psychiatric history. A differential should be presented and discussed briefly, followed by initial plans and prognosis.

The formulation should start with a brief sentence that summarizes the case. You should also include the family and personal history relevant to the current situation, along with a medical and psychiatric history, including previous diagnoses of personality disorders. Mention previous hospitalizations and failed treatment regimens. Summarize the recent workup, including ancillary testing and labs. Present your diagnosis of each DSM-IV axis,

TABLE 14-2

Mental Status Exam Features Common to Borderline Personality Disorder

Mental Status Exam	Features
Appearance	May have multiple cuts on arms
Behavior	Marked impulsivity
Speech	Normal
Affect	Rapid changes in affect from very happy to very sad
Thought process	Logical
Thought content	Reasonable
Perceptions	Intact
Cognition	Intact
Consciousness	Normal
Oriented	Difficulty with one's own identity
Memory	Intact
Judgment	Normal
Insight	Usually poor; feels misunderstood

focusing on axes I and II. An example formulation for this case patient is as follows:

The patient is a 31-year-old single woman with a difficult upbringing, including repeated sexual assault by a stepfather since the age of 8. She has never really known her biologic father, and she has a strained relationship with her mother. The patient had numerous early sexual experiences and some 50 sexual partners in her life, all heterosexual. She notes that she falls in love fast, but then quickly becomes "tired" of her boyfriends and dumps them. She started self-cutting with a razor at age 13. She describes no long-lasting relationships and reports feeling "empty and dull" inside. She first saw a psychiatrist at the age of 8, and since then, she has been in treatment with 15 different psychiatrists and 10 different therapists. She reports that several of the male providers had confessed their love to her, and when she did not reciprocate, they discharged her from their services (not confirmed by an outside informant). She has been diagnosed with major depressive disorder, bipolar affective disorder type II and later type I, panic disorder, generalized anxiety disorder, Personality disorder not otherwise specified, and borderline personality disorder. She has been on numerous psychiatric medications, including Prozac, Zoloft, Lexapro, Wellbutrin, lithium, Abilify, Zyprexa, Risperdal, Haldol, Ativan, and Valium. She describes adequate trials of these medications, although there are no records at this time to support this. She reports that none of these medications have helped with her symptoms. She has been admitted to psychiatric units six times in her life and describes six prior suicide attempts by cutting her wrists and overdosing on psychiatric medications. She is unable to provide a clear history of sustained disturbance in mood that last for a week or more and denies a history of substance abuse. Her urine toxicology was negative. Given the above history, the patient is being formulated with mood disorder not otherwise specified until further information from a collateral informant is obtained. There is also a strong likelihood that she has borderline personality disorder, although this diagnosis should also be provisional until a more thorough evaluation is completed.

Treatment

The treatment of personality disorders involves psychotherapy and medication. Personality disorders are some of the most difficult disorders to treat because patients do not easily open up with their therapists and the criticism they perceive tends to cause them to experience feelings of anger and alienation. Those who maintain their relationships with their therapist over many years are the most likely to succeed.

There are many different approaches to psychotherapy. Some focus on the emotions underlying personality disorders, and others try to reinforce certain behaviors and coping mechanisms. Each approach has its pros and cons, and often patients may try different approaches with their therapist. For borderline personality disorder specifically, a certain type of behavioral psychotherapy called *dialectic behavioral therapy* concentrates on the patient's observing feelings without reacting to them, allowing the patient to take control of his or her emotions.

Medical therapy depends on other comorbidities, such as major depression and anxiety disorders, which often accompany personality disorders. Patients with personality disorders are often treated with selective serotonin reuptake inhibitors to relieve symptoms of depression (see Treatment section of Chapter 12) and anxiety (see Treatment section of Chapter 15). Anxiolytics are addictive and should be avoided if possible. For compulsive behaviors related to personality disorders, anticonvulsants are commonly prescribed; for those with distorted thinking, antipsychotic medication (see Treatment section of Chapter 13) may prove beneficial. Details about the scope of these medications and their side effects can be found in the chapters of this book related to their respective disorders.

EXTENDED INHOSPITAL MANAGEMENT

The primary team should see the patient on rounds each morning and perform a tailored MSE, focusing on her subset of symptoms. For patients with borderline personality disorder, alert all members of the team to beware of splitting (the patient will idealize certain staff members and devalue others because she sees the world in black and white). Splitting may also occur within the same individual, so that the patient may initially shower you with compliments and then make you out to be uncaring or incompetent. For these reasons, it is particularly important to maintain your professional boundaries.

CLINICAL PEARL

Give your patient the treatment he or she needs, but do not give any special treatment relative to other patients.

DISPOSITION

Discharge Goals

The patient should be discharged when she reports improvement of mood toward baseline, denies suicidal ideation, and describes a calmer state. Refer the patient to an individual therapist for weekly therapy and/or to a dialectic behavioral therapy (DBT) group in her area.

Outpatient Care

The patient should have outpatient follow-up arranged prior to discharge. If she is on medications, she should follow up with a psychiatrist. If she is not on medications, she may follow up with a therapist alone.

WHAT YOU NEED TO REMEMBER

- Personality disorders are pervasive disorders of character styles that produce impairment in relationships and career. Personality disorders, along with mental retardation, are coded on axis II, unlike other psychiatric diseases, such as mood disorders, schizophrenia, and substance abuse, which are coded on axis I.
- There are three main clusters of personality disorders:
    A: Odd and eccentric. Includes paranoid, schizoid, and schizotypal personality disorders

B: Dramatic. Includes histrionic, narcissistic, borderline personality, and antisocial personality disorders

C: Anxious. Includes avoidant, dependent, and obsessive-compulsive personality disorders

- A good psychiatric history is key to proper diagnosis and treatment. The MSE is the psychiatrist's version of the internist's physical examination and is critical for assessment and diagnosis. As a medical student, the most important part of your presentation to the attending is perhaps the MSE.
- The treatment of personality disorders involves psychotherapy and medication.

REFERENCE

1. Grant BF, Hasin DS, Stinson FS, et al. Prevalence, correlates, and disability of personality disorders in the United States: results from the national epidemiologic survey on alcohol and related conditions. *J Clin Psychiatry* 2004;65(7):948–958.

SUGGESTED READINGS

Cummings JL, Mega MS. *Neuropsychiatry and Behavioral Neuroscience*. Oxford, UK: Oxford University Press, 2003.

Frances AJ, Ross R. *Diagnostic and Statistical Manual of Mental Disorders (DSM-IV-TR)*. 4th Ed text rev. Arlington, VA: American Psychiatric Association, 2003.

Gabbard GO. *Psychodynamic Psychiatry in Clinical Practice*. 3rd Ed. Arlington, VA: American Psychiatry Press, 2000.

Johnson SM. *Character Styles*. New York: WW Norton and Company, 1994.

Kaufman DM. *Clinical Neurology for Psychiatrists*. Philadelphia: WB Saunders, 2006.

McWilliams N. *Psychoanalytic Diagnosis: Understanding Personality Structure in the Clinical Process*. New York: The Guilford Press, 1994.

Tomb DA. *House Officer Series: Psychiatry*. 6th Ed. Philadelphia: Lippincott Williams & Wilkins, 1999.

Yudofsky SC. *Fatal Flaws: Navigating Destructive Relationships with People with Disorders of Personality and Character*. Arlington, VA5: American Psychiatric Publishing, 2005.

Anxiety Disorders

THE PATIENT ENCOUNTER

A 22-year-old man with no significant past cardiac history presents to the emergency department (ED) with complaints of his heart "pounding," sweating, shortness of breath, nausea, and feeling "like I'm going to die" that has been occurring intermittently for the past 2 months and getting worse. His parents were concerned there was something wrong with his heart so they brought him to the emergency room. During the interview, the man admits that he used to have panic attacks as a teenager. The cardiac workup is thus far unremarkable, and a psychiatry consult is called.

OVERVIEW

Definition and Pathophysiology

Anxiety is a normal response to stress. But if the anxiety is overwhelming or disabling, or when anxiety is provoked abnormally in a nonstressful situation, the anxiety becomes a disorder. There are five major types of anxiety disorder, which are listed in Table 15-1.

- *Generalized anxiety disorder.* Generalized anxiety disorder is an inclusive diagnosis for patients who experience uncomfortable levels of anxiety under normal daily circumstances.
- *Obsessive-compulsive disorder.* Obsessive-compulsive disorder (OCD) is fairly recognizable as an uncontrollable urge to perform repetitive behaviors (compulsions) or think certain thoughts (obsessions) that compromise daily activities. Anxiety develops when the patient is involved in situations in which the behaviors cannot be done and the obsessions are overwhelming. For example, a patient with obsessive-compulsive disorder may avoid germs by washing his hands frequently. However, if a sink is not available to wash his hands, the patient may develop severe anxiety because of obsessions about the germs on his hands.
- *Panic disorder.* Panic disorder is reserved for those who have unexplained transient episodes of severe anxiety with physical symptoms such as sweating, hyperventilation, and chest pain. The distinction between generalized

TABLE 15-1
Anxiety Disorders

Disorder	Features
Generalized anxiety disorder	Anxiety that is chronically provoked by nonstressful situations
Obsessive-compulsive disorder	Recurrent unwanted thoughts (obsessions) or repetitive behaviors (compulsions) that provoke anxiety if not performed
Panic disorder	Intermittent and unexpected bouts of severe anxiety accompanied by physical symptoms
Posttraumatic stress disorder	Anxiety that develops after a psychologically traumatic event
Social anxiety disorder	Anxiety limited to one social situation, such as public speaking

anxiety disorder and panic disorder is important because they can be treated differently.

- *Posttraumatic stress disorder.* Posttraumatic stress disorder (PTSD) may initially present as generalized anxiety disorder or panic disorder, but a carefully taken patient history will often reveal a recurring trigger of memory or physical symptoms of a previously experienced psychologically traumatizing event.

- *Social anxiety disorder.* Social anxiety disorder is the mildest of the anxiety disorders. It includes patients who develop anxiety about being in social situations, ranging from public speaking to agoraphobia (fear of leaving home).

Anxiety disorders impact society in many different ways. For example, individuals with panic disorder are five to seven times more likely to highly use medical services than those without panic disorder. Anxiety disorders are also associated with significant impairments in physical and psychosocial function, as well as quality of life. They are associated with increased rates of substance abuse, marital and work problems, and suicide attempts.

The pathophysiology of anxiety disorders is not well understood. The traditional teaching is that patients with anxiety disorders have an overactive sympathetic system that responds inappropriately to benign stimuli.

CLINICAL PEARL

On the neurotransmitter level, it is thought that anxiety disorders arise out of an imbalance of too little serotonergic activity plus overactive noradrenergic activity. These theories are oversimplifications of a complicated behavioral process that likely includes genetic predispositions and environmental stressors.

Epidemiology

All together, anxiety disorders have a 20% lifetime prevalence in the U.S. population. They have a bimodal onset among individuals 15 to 24 years old, and a second onset among individuals aged 45 to 54. First-degree relatives of patients with anxiety disorders have up to an eightfold increased risk of developing an anxiety disorder.

ACUTE MANAGEMENT AND WORKUP

The presentation of an acute anxiety attack is very similar to an acute coronary syndrome, including chest pain and shortness of breath. The primary concern of the emergency staff is to rule out a life-threatening or medically dangerous condition, such as coronary artery disease and pneumonia. As with any presentation of chest pain, the initial assessment should focus on ruling out a cardiac cause. Emergency department staff are quite adept at cardiac workups, but before pursuing a psychiatric workup, quickly look through the patient's chart, paying particular attention to his vital signs, and then make sure he is stable. Even though you are being called to deal with a possible psychiatric situation, be vigilant for clues of nonpsychiatric presentations of chest pain, including cardiac, pulmonary, neurologic, and hematologic causes.

The First 15 Minutes

Patients with an acute panic attack or anxiety exacerbation feel like they are about to die. Be reassured—they are not. The goal of the first 15 minutes in evaluating a patient with anxiety disorder is to confirm the diagnosis and rule out other nonpsychiatric medical conditions, such as myocardial infarction. You do not want to miss an important life-threatening condition even in a patient with a known history of anxiety disorder; thus each patient deserves a good general medical workup in addition to psychiatric care for anxiety.

Initial Assessment

For acute anxiety attacks, the first goal is to calm the patient down to allow for a complete medical workup, including a cardiac workup. Toward that end, reassure your patient that you and the emergency room staff are doing everything you and they can to help him. Some patients will feel better knowing that many people are involved in their care, whereas others may get more anxious by the bustle of the staff around them. In that case, try to reduce the noise (especially false alarms from cardiac monitors) and minimize anxiety-provoking activity around your patient. In a patient with anxiety-related respiratory distress, ensure your patient is on room air pulse oximetry and the O_2 saturation is within normal limits (97%–99% for most patients, although smokers may have a lower O_2 saturation); for a hyperventilating patient, have him rebreathe in a paper bag at a breathing rate of <20 breaths per minute. After your patient calms down, reassess his vital signs for an expected reduction in heart rate and blood pressure. If your patient is truly inconsolable and cannot calm down, or if he appears unusually agitated, intoxicated, disoriented, or is actively trying to harm himself, order an observer (sitter or security guard). In special circumstances in which the anxiety is preventing your patient's ability to function, consider administering 1 to 2 mg of lorazepam by mouth or intramuscularly if he is unmanageable and refuses medications by mouth.

Send for labs, including complete blood count (CBC) with differential, complete metabolic panel (CMP), blood toxicology (alcohol level), urine drug screen (amphetamines, cocaine, and phencyclidine), urinalysis, and thyroid function tests. You should also order an electrocardiogram (ECG) to rule out cardiac complications if this has not already been ordered. Chest radiography is useful to rule out other causes of chest pain with dyspnea. An electroencephalogram (EEG) may also be helpful if his history is suspicious for seizure activity (partial complex seizures can manifest anxiety as aura and ictal phenomena). Partial seizures tend to be much shorter than panic attacks, which can last up to 60 minutes.

Be vigilant for atypical presentations of emergent conditions that can present with anxiety, including myocardial infarction and pulmonary embolism. With a high index of suspicion, you may consider cardiac enzymes (if you suspect acute coronary syndrome) and a D-dimer assay (to exclude a pulmonary embolism). In patients who may be at high risk for a pulmonary embolus, order appropriate testing, such as ventilation/perfusion (V/Q) scanning, duplex ultrasonography, spiral CT scanning, pulmonary angiography, or multidetector CT angiography if available.

Once you have determined the patient is stable, you can begin your psychiatric workup.

Admission Criteria and Level of Care Criteria

Patients with uncomplicated panic disorder will not usually require admission to the hospital. However, anxiety disorders are frequently comorbid with depressive disorders, so be sure to screen for suicidal ideation. Those who have positive test results on any of several of the previously mentioned medical tests may require hospitalization to an intensive care unit (ICU) or medical setting for further workup to rule out medical causes (i.e., myocar-dial infarction [MI], pulmonary embolism, seizure disorder) with a psychi-atric consult. Notify the admitting team that the psychiatry service will fol-low the patient closely and reassess his need for inpatient psychiatric treatment after his medical workup (or rule out) is complete.

There are cases of emergent medical complications secondary to the phobic fears (e.g., fear of swallowing, which leads to dehydration and weight loss), imminent loss of job or relationship, inability to undergo necessary medical procedures, risk of children's welfare, or acute and rapid generaliza-tion of phobic behavior. In such cases, mobilization of family resources or high-potency benzodiazepines may be the starting point for treatment once the patient has received basic educational information.

Patients with anxiety disorder should be admitted to an inpatient psychi-atric unit if they are medically stable and require 24-hour nursing or obser-vation, are unable to care for themselves outside of the hospital, or it is antic-ipated that intensive medication changes will occur over a short period of time. Patients who lack capacity to sign a voluntary form or who are in imminent danger of hurting themselves or others should be involuntarily committed.

The First 24 Hours

The history is key to evaluating the psychiatric patient. Obtain what infor-mation you can in the ER and complete the initial workup on the floor.

History

Key elements of the history that you should obtain are the following:

- *Family history.* Obtaining the patient's family history will help you deter-mine genetic loading. For example, first-degree relatives of individuals with panic disorder are seven times more likely to also have panic disor-der. Anxiety disorders are associated with an increased risk of suicide. A family history of suicide is itself a risk factor for suicide in an individual.
- *Personal history.* In psychiatric evaluations, understanding the patient's personal history is critical for a thorough assessment. In the short term, be sure to cover his social circumstances (i.e., finances, legal problems, employment, current social supports/relationships, dependents, and hous-ing) as these may have the most immediate bearing on panic symptoms. A more complete personal history may be obtained after admission to the floor; you should ask about a history of past relationships, as well as the patient's educational background, abuse history, childhood development, and childhood personality. Obtain a brief legal history, including any total jail time, violent arrests, and pending legal issues. Although patients may attempt to avoid jail by seeking hospitalization, it must also be considered that the fear of incarceration may be a significant stressor.

- *Substance abuse history.* For every substance, ask the patient how much and how often he uses, his first use, his most recent use, the route of administration, and whether he has had withdrawal signs or symptoms. In establishing the patient's substance abuse history, ask about cigarettes, alcohol, caffeine, and street drugs (diazepam, clonazepam, cocaine, and other stimulants.) Ask about his pattern and origin of usage. It is not uncommon for patients with social anxiety to self-medicate before social gatherings. Document any prior history of substance abuse treatment. Try to get a history for the patient's symptoms during periods of abstinence from drugs. This will be important in deciding whether the patient has a prior anxiety disorder, substance-induced panic disorder, or is self-medicating his symptoms.
- *Past psychiatric history.* Ask the patient if he has a psychiatrist or takes any psychiatric medications. Obtain information regarding the patient's premorbid (or baseline) personality and the onset of his first anxiety symptoms. Get a description of a typical anxiety episode. Inquire about phobias, triggers, and relieving factors. In addition, ask about recurrent thoughts, impulses, or images that are intrusive, knowingly inappropriate, and cause anxiety. These thoughts may also be met with repeated attempts to ignore or suppress them. When assessing posttraumatic stress disorder (PTSD), ask about a history of actual or threatened death, serious injury, or a threat to the physical well-being of oneself or others. This seems elementary but is often overlooked.
- *History of the present illness.* Find out what brought your patient to the hospital today. You will want to determine how fast the symptoms began. Panic disorder typically begins suddenly and peaks within 10 to 15 minutes and can last up to an hour. Be sure to ask about any potential triggering factors, such as illness, childbirth, trauma, loss, or external stressors. Find out if this is the first episode or one in a lifetime series of episodes. Be sure to ask if he thinks the anxiety, fear, or obsession is excessive (ego-dystonic) or in harmony with his self-image (ego-syntonic.) Most psychiatric evaluations will require you to formally assess the risk of suicide and dangerousness as well as any protective factors.

Physical Examination

Among anxiety disorders, the two you will most commonly see in the hospital are general anxiety disorder and panic disorder. Below is an example of the mental status exam (MSE) for our patient with generalized anxiety disorder:

> *The patient was a 22-year-old white man who appeared his stated age. He was slightly overweight, neatly groomed, and wearing dress clothes with his tie hanging loosely around his neck. He sat on the side of the bed and frequently visually scanned the room. He was visibly more anxious when others entered*

the room during the interview; he carefully watched them and often asked if he was all right. He was diaphoretic and breathing rapidly. During the interview, he was fidgety but without stereotypical movements. His speech was normal in volume and amount, but he was occasionally breathless. Several times, he asked if he was having a heart attack and stated that he felt like "something was wrong." His thought process was logical and linear but preoccupied with his symptoms. He denied any suicidal or homicidal ideation. He had no prior history of suicide and is currently employed and happily married. Though he does have some excessive worry regarding the future, he has a relatively low risk of suicide. He denied any auditory or visual hallucinations and did not exhibit any signs of thought disorder. He described his mood as "just scared something is really wrong with me." His affect was anxious but stable and was congruent with his stated mood. His intelligence was above average based on his vocabulary, abstraction abilities, general information, and educational achievement. He was alert and oriented and received a score of 29/30 on his MMSE [Mini-Mental Status Exam], missing one point for recall after 5 minutes.

TABLE 15-2
Mental Status Exam Features Common to Anxiety Disorders

Mental Status Exam	Features
Appearance	Facial expressions of anxiety and panic
Behavior	Fidgety and hyperactive
Speech	Interrupted by hyperventilation
Affect	Irritability, impatience
Thought process	Logical
Thought content	Normal
Perceptions	Derealization, sense of doom
Cognition	Difficulty concentrating
Consciousness	Hyperalert
Oriented	Intact
Memory	Poor working memory
Judgment	Reasonable
Insight	Usually good insight

Table 15-2 lists the mental status exam features that are common in anxiety disorders.

Labs and Tests to Consider

Although the patient is likely to have been medically cleared in the ER, you want to ensure common medical causes of anxiety have been ruled out. It is standard to check levels of thyroid-stimulating hormone (TSH) and B12, as well as CBC and CMP. Toxicology, including blood alcohol and urine drug screen, is especially important because of the high comorbidity of substance abuse in anxiety disorders (Table 15-3). Cardiovascular illness can present with a pattern of symptoms that resemble anxiety disorders, so you will want to ensure an ECG and a measure of cardiac enzymes have been done (Table 15-4). In patients presenting with atypical symptoms suggestive of seizure activity, including a short duration of attack (usually 1 to 2 minutes), motor automatisms, age >45 years at onset of attacks, a history of febrile convulsions, and lack of response to conventional treatments for panic attacks, check an EEG.

Assessment

Anxiety has multiple causes that may require investigation, depending on the patient's presentation. An accurate diagnosis of anxiety disorders, and, in

TABLE 15-3
Key Laboratory Tests and Rationales for Testing

Test	Rationale
Heme-8 with differential	Rule out (r/o) leukocytosis associated with infection
Complete metabolic panel	R/o evidence of metabolic dysfunction such as acute renal failure/uremia, electrolyte imbalance such as hyperkalemia.
Urine toxicity screen	R/o drug and alcohol intoxication
Thyroid-stimulating hormone (TSH)	R/o hyperthyroidism/hypothyroidism
Cardiac enzymes (troponins, creatine kinase [CK])	R/o acute myocardial infarction

TABLE 15-4
Key Ancillary Tests and Rationales for Testing

Test	Rationale
Electrocardiogram (ECG)	Rule out acute myocardial infarction and arrythmias
Electroencephalogram (EEG)	Evaluate for spikes or sharp waves (seizure activity) or diffuse cerebral slowing (altered mental status)

particular, panic disorder, is important because these patients use the ED at a higher rate and are at risk for unnecessary procedures. Nonpsychiatric causes of anxiety must be excluded first (Table 15-5).

For the patient in the initial case study, the formulation might read as follows:

> *This is a 22-year-old while man who was recently (2 weeks ago) passed over for a promotion at work. This is his third episode of severe anxiety in the past 6 months, during which he experiences tachycardia, diaphoresis, shortness of breath, nausea, intense anxiety, and a feeling of dread. The last episode was 1 week ago, and since that time he has become concerned he was going to have a heart attack. He also reported a prior episode of depression 5 years ago that was successfully treated with a selective serotonin reuptake inhibitor (SSRI). The patient described his mother as "a worrier" and has a maternal family history of alcoholism. He has worked for the same company for 2 years and felt that he deserved a promotion. He denied drug or alcohol use but does have several cups of coffee throughout*

TABLE 15-5
Nonpsychiatric Causes of Anxiety

Substance Use	Cardiopulmonary	Neurologic	Systemic
Alcohol withdrawal	Myocardial ischemia	Epilepsy	Thyroid disease
Decongestants	Arrhythmias	Migraine	Hypoglycemia
Asthma medications	Hypoxia	Huntington disease	Pheochromo-cytoma
Caffeine		Brain tumor	Porphyria

the day. This episode of anxiety was likely exacerbated by recent stressors at work and complicated by his caffeine intake and possible family history of anxiety. Given the presentation of his symptoms and that he has been ruled out for MI, he is being formulated with panic disorder without agoraphobia. He would likely benefit from medication management together with cognitive behavioral therapy. Inpatient psychiatric admission is not recommended at this time because he has been ruled out for emergent medical problems and his anxiety has significantly abated after he received 2 mg of Ativan PO on admission to the ED. Reinitiation of an SSRI should be considered in this patient. He will be scheduled for follow-up in the outpatient clinic for medication management and individual psychotherapy.

Treatment

Generalized anxiety disorder tends to be chronic with a fluctuating course. It responds well to both pharmacologic and cognitive behavioral treatments, with the greatest improvement from a combination of both modalities. SSRIs are the first-line medication in the treatment of generalized anxiety disorder, PTSD, and obsessive-compulsive disorder because of their excellent safety profile and efficacy. However, SSRIs have the potential to cause initial restlessness and increased anxiety, so patients must be educated about these potential phenomena. Although SSRIs have shown good efficacy in the treatment of anxiety disorders, they have a slow onset that often requires patients to wait 3 to 6 weeks for symptoms to improve.

Benzodiazepines are frequently used for the rapid treatment of both generalized anxiety disorder and panic disorder because of their efficacy and rapid onset. The potential for abuse and dependence must be considered before prescribing benzodiazepines, although a history of substance abuse is not an absolute contraindication to benzodiazepine treatment. Long-term therapy is generally achieved with SSRIs (see Treatment section of Chapter 12 for details about this drug class).

Cognitive behavioral therapy (CBT) is helpful for treatment of all types of anxiety disorders because it addresses catastrophic misinterpretations and somatic sensations as well as helping the patient to eliminate avoidant behavior. CBT is typically time limited, with only 12 to 15 sessions. CBT includes educational interventions, cognitive restructuring, exposure interventions, and anxiety management skills.

EXTENDED INHOSPITAL MANAGEMENT

The primary team should see the patient on rounds each morning and perform a tailored MSE that focuses on his subset of symptoms. For patients with anxiety, ask about mood, passive death wishes, suicidal and homicidal ideation, paranoia, and sequelae of panic disorder, including

CLINICAL PEARL

Panic disorder responds to SSRI treatment in 60% to 70% of cases. SSRIs require 3 to 6 weeks before beneficial effects are noted. For immediate treatment of symptoms, benzodiazepines may be used.

depersonalization and derealization. While the patient is hospitalized, start him on an SSRI.

While the patient is in the hospital, you can provide brief informational explanations about the nature of the patient's panic disorder, including educating the patient about the somatic sensations that occur during panic attacks. Address any comorbid substance abuse or dependence and provide withdrawal management as needed.

DISPOSITION

Discharge Goals

As in all psychiatric discharges, the patient may go home when he is stable in the disease course and no longer poses a threat to himself or others. He must be able to take care of himself, and there must be reasonable confidence that the patient will continue to do well outside of the hospital and on his own. The particular goals of an admission for anxiety disorder include the following:

• Exclusion of emergent and medical causes of anxiety
• Treatment for substance abuse and/or withdrawal
• Discussion with the patient and his family about the nature of his somatic symptoms and self-perpetuating patterns that may serve to maintain the disorder. It may also be helpful to provide some initial exposure to anxiety management skills (i.e., muscle relaxation training).

Outpatient Care

The patient should have outpatient follow-up arranged prior to discharge. Ideally, follow-up should be provided by a psychiatrist for both pharmacotherapy and cognitive behavioral therapy as the combination of these treatments is likely to provide a better outcome for patients than medical treatment alone. If the cause was determined to be medical or neurologic, follow-up should be arranged with the patient's primary care physician or neurologist.

WHAT YOU NEED TO REMEMBER

- Anxiety disorder is a disabling, anxious response to stimuli or an abnormally anxious response to a nonstressful situation.
- Acute presentations of anxiety attacks can mimic cardiac and pulmonary causes of chest pain, shortness of breath, and diaphoresis.
- Before making the diagnosis an acute anxiety attack, all medical causes should be ruled out.
- Obtaining a thorough patient history is important in distinguishing among the five major types of anxiety disorders.
- Medical therapy and cognitive behavioral psychotherapies are the standards of treatment for patients with anxiety disorders.

SUGGESTED READINGS

Cohen Bruce J. *Theory and Practice of Psychiatry*. Oxford, UK: Oxford University Press, 2003.

Frances AJ, Ross R. *Diagnostic and Statistical Manual of Mental Disorders (DSM-IV-TR)*. 4th Ed text rev. Arlington, VA: American Psychiatric Association, 2003.

Hales RE, Yudofsky SC. *Essentials of Clinical Psychiatry*. Arlington, VA: American Psychiatry Publishing, 2004.

Kaufman DM. *Clinical Neurology for Psychiatrists*. Philadelphia: WB Saunders, 2006.

Stern TA, Fricchione GL, Cassem NH, et al. *Massachusetts General Hospital Handbook of General Hospital Psychiatry*. St. Louis: Mosby, 2004.

Tomb DA. *House Officer Series: Psychiatry*. 6th Ed. Philadelphia: Lippincott Williams & Wilkins, 1999.

Index

Page numbers followed by f indicate figure; those followed by t indicate table.

Vitamin deficiencies
  alcoholism and, 105
  gait disorders and, 111
  numbness and tingling in, 80
Voice, hoarseness, 10

W
Walking
  assessment of, 119
  festination, 104
  pain during, 104
  in patients with dizziness, 119
  process of, 101
  shortness of breath during, 104
Wallenberg syndrome, 132
Water, X-ray attenuation, 17t
Weakness
  acute management, 51–60
    admission criteria, 52
    initial assessment, 51–52
    level of care criteria, 52
  assessments
    ancillary testing, 56
    components of, 56–60
    imaging, 56, 57t
    laboratory tests, 55–56, 56t
    mental status, 54–55
    patient history, 53–54
    physical examination, 54–55
  asymmetric, in seizure patients, 91
  below neck, spinal cord lesions and, 2
  brainstem lesions and, 2
  definition, 48–51
  differential diagnoses, 60, 61t–64t
  disposition

discharge goals, 68
  outpatient care, 68–69
epidemiology of, 51
extended inhospital management, 60
focal, 48, 52
in gait disorders, 105
generalized, 48
ipsilateral face/contralateral body, 2
lesion localization, 3t
localization of, 53–54
one sided, 1
pathophysiology of, 48–51
patient encounters, 48
postictal, 61t
subcortical white matter lesions and, 1
treatment, 60
Wellbutrin, side effects of, 191
Wernicke area, language and, 168–169
White matter
  dementias and, 169
  lesions localized to, 1–2
  X-ray attenuation, 17t
Wilson disease, psychotic symptoms in, 201
Wrist extension, assessment of, 11
Wrist flexion, assessment of, 11

X
X-rays
  after falls, 102
  attenuation in Hounsfield units, 17t
  plain film, 23

Z
Zonisamide (Zonegran), 99t